Medical Biochemistry at a Glance

Dedication

In memory of Gordon Hartman (1936–2004), friend and colleague whose enthusiasm and encyclopaedic knowledge were an asset to all who knew him.

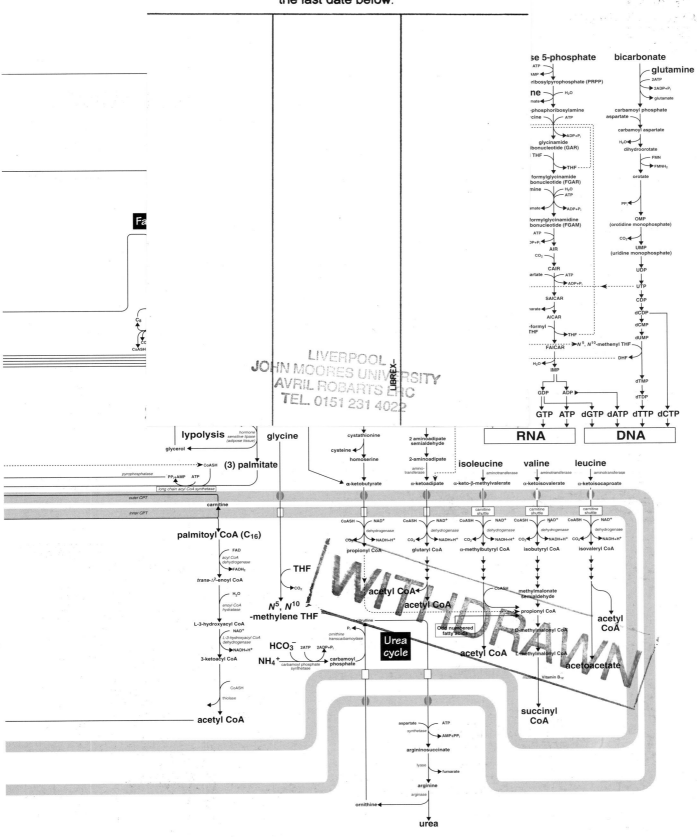

Medical Biochemistry at a Glance

Dr J. G. Salway

School of Biomedical and Molecular Sciences
University of Surrey
Guildford
Surrey, UK

Second edition

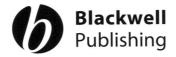

© 2006 J.G. Salway
Published by Blackwell Publishing Ltd
Blackwell Publishing, Inc., 350 Main Street, Malden, Massachusetts 02148-5020, USA
Blackwell Publishing Ltd, 9600 Garsington Road, Oxford OX4 2DQ, UK
Blackwell Publishing Asia Pty Ltd, 550 Swanston Street, Carlton, Victoria 3053, Australia

First published 1996
Second edition published 2006

3   2008

Library of Congress Cataloging-in-Publication Data

Salway, J. G.
    Medical biochemistry at a glance / J. G. Salway. — 2nd ed.
        p. ; cm.
    Rev. ed. of: Medical biochemistry at a glance / Ben Greenstein, Adam
Greenstein. 1996.
    Includes bibliographical references and index.
    ISBN: 978-1-4051-1322-9 (alk. paper)
    1. Biochemistry—Outlines, syllabi, etc. 2. Clinical biochemistry—Outlines, syllabi,
etc. I. Greenstein, Ben, 1941– . Medical biochemistry at a glance. II. Title. [DNLM: 1.
 Biochemistry. QU 4 S186m 2006]
    QP514.2.G76 2006
    612'.015—dc22
                                                                        2005025952

ISBN: 978-1-4051-1322-9

A catalogue record for this title is available from the British Library

Set in 9/11.5 Times by SNP Best-set Typesetter Ltd, Hong Kong
Printed and bound in India by Replika Press Pvt. Ltd

Commissioning Editor: Vicki Noyes, Martin Sugden
Editorial Assistant: Caroline Aders
Development Editor: Geraldine Jeffers
Production Controller: Kate Charman

For further information on Blackwell Publishing, visit our website:
http://www.blackwellpublishing.com

The publisher's policy is to use permanent paper from mills that operate a sustainable forestry policy,
and which has been manufactured from pulp processed using acid-free and elementary chlorine-free
practices. Furthermore, the publisher ensures that the text paper and cover board used have met
acceptable environmental accreditation standards.

Contents

Preface

Medical Biochemistry at a Glance is written for medical students and students of the biomedical sciences such as biochemists, medical laboratory scientists, veterinary scientists, dentists, pharmacologists, physiologists, physiotherapists, nutritionists, food scientists, nurses, medical physicists, microbiologists and students of sports science. This book aspires to present the subject of biochemistry relevant to students of medical science in the concise two-page format of the "At a Glance" series. The dictate of the series values brevity as a virtue so those aspects of biochemistry known as Molecular Biology are covered elsewhere in *Medical Genetics at a Glance*.

Students who study biochemistry as a subsidiary part of their course are frequently overwhelmed by the complexity and huge amount of detail involved. Lecturers will be familiar with the anxious expression of students as they complain "*How much of this do we need to know?*" or "*Do we need to memorise all the structural formulae and the chemical reactions?*" In fairness, biochemistry **is** a complex and heavily detailed subject. Students should have two objectives: (i) **to study and understand** biochemical concepts and reactions but not necessarily memorise the structural details, and

(ii) **to prepare for examinations** by determining the amount of detail required by intelligent perusal of lecture notes and past examination papers.

Medical Biochemistry at a Glance is written with these two objectives in mind. Judicious study of the comprehensive metabolic chart on the inside cover and the detailed chart on the back inside cover featuring formulae and enzymes catalysing the reaction will enable an understanding of metabolic biochemistry.

However, in the text of the book, complex detail is subjugated to a faint background so as to emphasise the most important aspect of the topic. However, students must familiarise themselves with the requirements of their particular examination board to determine how much they should trust to memory.

Finally, the inspiration for *Medical Biochemistry at a Glance* has developed from *Metabolism at a Glance* which I wrote in 1994 and is now in its third edition. The latter is a more advanced book but the similarity of style between these two books facilitates progression to a higher level by students specialising in metabolism and disorders of metabolism.

Acknowledgements

I have been very encouraged by the support of colleagues and I appreciate their advice and encouragement during the preparation of this book. I am particularly grateful to: Loranne Agius, Wynne Aherne, Beatrice Evans, Martyn Egerton, George Elder, Janet Brown, Neil Dalton, John Findlay, Keith Frayn, Geoffrey Gibbons, Anna Gloyn, Barry Gould, Bruce Griffin, Stephen Halloran, James Hooper, Marie Jackson, Garry John, John Lodge, Chris O'Callaghan, Robert Robergs, Ann Saada, Marie Skerry, John Stafford, Andrew Symons, John Wright and Richard Veech. Once again my gratitude is due to Rosemary James for her advice and encouragement and for casting her eagle eye over the typescript. I am most grateful to Fiona Goodgame of Blackwell Publishing for commissioning this book, to Vicki Noyes who negotiated all the resources I needed, and to their successor Martin Sugden for editorial guidance. I have been very fortunate to have the patient support of Geraldine Jeffers throughout the production process and of Mirjana Misina during the final stages as project manager. The excellent, comprehensive index was compiled by Philip Aslett. Finally I would especially like to acknowledge the collaboration with Elaine Leggett of Oxford Designers and Illustrators who has drawn the artwork from my primitive sketches. Such is the complexity of the artwork that I would not have contemplated this work without the assurance of Elaine's help, so it is true to say that without Elaine's support this book would not have been published.

Inevitably omissions and errors will have occurred and I would be most grateful to have these drawn to my attention.

J. G. Salway
Chiddingfold
Surrey, UK
March 2005
j.salway@btinternet.com

Figure Key

 Therapeutic drug

 Disease or poison

 Associated with diagnostic blood test

 Excretion in urine or faeces. Product may be used in diagnosis

 SAM (S-adenosylmethionine) A methyl donor

 Currently the subject of research, debate or clinical trials

 Currently the subject of research, debate or clinical trials

 Fed-state or dietary intake

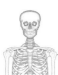 Fasting state, starvation

 Pathway operates in cardiac muscle

 Pathway operates in skeletal muscle

 Pathway operates in liver

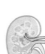 Pathway operates in kidney

 A hydrophobic group

 A hydrophilic group

cyclic AMP

inactive protein kinase A → **active protein kinase A**

PKA (protein kinase A) is activated by cyclic AMP which binds to and removes the regulatory (inhibiting) subunits.

 Insulin receptor is activated by autophosphorylation of the β-subunits when insulin binds to the α-subunits

 IRS-1 (Insulin Receptor Substrate-1).

 P85. 85kDa protein is regulatory subunit of PI-3 kinase. Links IRS-1 to PI-3 kinase

 PI-3 kinase. Phosphorylates the 3-hydroxyl group of PIP2 to form phosphatidylinositol 3,4,5-trisphosphate

 AKT (previously known as PKB). A serine/threonine protein kinase. Binds to PIP3.

 PDK-1. Phosphoinositide Dependent Kinase-1 is activated by phosphatidylinositol 3,4,5-trisphosphate

 Glycogen Synthase Kinase -3. Constitutively active in fasting state. Is inhibited when phosphorylated by AKT

 Protein phosphatase-1. Activated by insulin-generated signals

SI/Mass Unit Conversions

Total bilirubin

< 20 μMol/L $\xrightarrow{(\times 17.1)}$ $\xleftarrow{(\div 17.1)}$ < 1.2 mg/dL

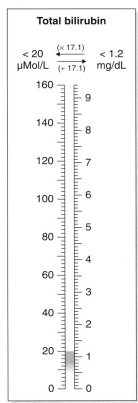

Calcium

2.0–2.5 mMol/L $\xrightarrow{(\times 0.25)}$ $\xleftarrow{(\div 0.25)}$ 8–10 mg/dL

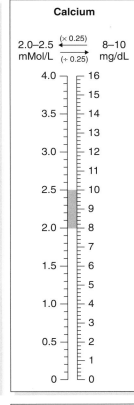

Creatinine

60–120 μMol/L $\xrightarrow{(\times 88.4)}$ $\xleftarrow{(\div 88.4)}$ 0.6–1.3 mg/dL

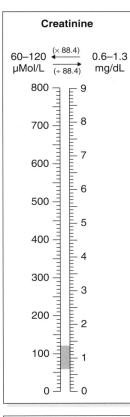

Glucose

< 6.0 mMol/L $\xrightarrow{(\times 0.056)}$ $\xleftarrow{(\div 0.056)}$ < 110 mg/dL

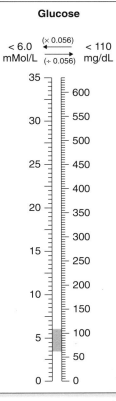

[H⁺]

(pH 7.35–7.45)   (35–45 nMol/L)

pH = $-\log_{10}$ [H⁺] in Moles
eg 100nMol/L
= $-\log_{10}$ 0.0000001 = pH 7.0

eg antilog$_{10}$ of −7.4 = 0.000000040 Mol/L
= 40 nMol/L

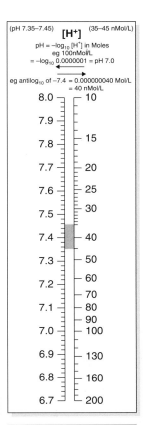

Phosphate / Phosphorus

0.6–1.25 mMol/L $\xrightarrow{(\times 0.323)}$ $\xleftarrow{(\div 0.323)}$ 1.9–3.9 mg/dL

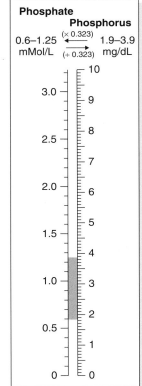

Thyroxine (T4)

7.25 pMol/L $\xrightarrow{(\times 12.87)}$ $\xleftarrow{(\div 12.87)}$ 0.5–2.0 ng/dL

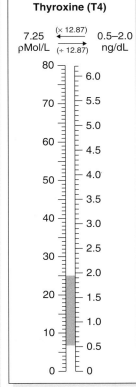

Triglycerides

target < 1.5 mMol/L $\xrightarrow{(\times 0.0113)}$ $\xleftarrow{(\div 0.0113)}$ target < 133 mg/dL

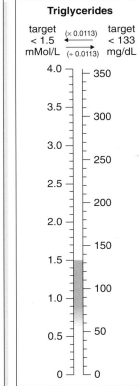

Urea / BUN

3–7 mMol/L $\xrightarrow{(\times 0.357)}$ $\xleftarrow{(\div 0.357)}$ 8–20 mg/dL

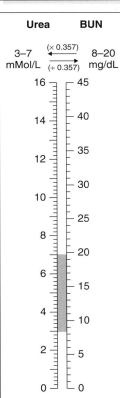

Total cholesterol

target < 4.0 mMol/L $\xrightarrow{(\times 0.0259)}$ $\xleftarrow{(\div 0.0259)}$ target < 155 mg/dL

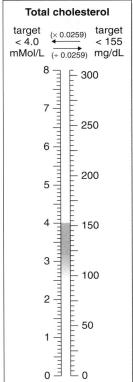

Acids, bases and hydrogen ions (protons)

Definition of pH

pH is defined as "*the negative logarithm to the base 10 of the hydrogen ion concentration*",

$pH = -\log_{10}[H^+]$

For example, at pH 7.0, the hydrogen ion concentration is 0.0000001 mMoles/L or 10^{-7} mMol/L.

The $\log_{10}$ of 0.0000001 is −7.0

Therefore, the negative $\log_{10}$ is −(−7.0) i.e. +7.0 and hence the pH is 7.0.

$$10,000 \times 100,000 = 1,000,000,000 = 10^9$$
$$\text{or}$$
$$10^4 \times 10^5 = 10^9$$
(adding powers is the same as multiplying the original number)

$$\text{Log}\ \frac{x}{y} = \log x - \log y$$

$$\text{Log}\ \frac{1}{x} = -\log x$$

Figure 1.1 Revision of logarithms.

Number	Equivalent as 10 to the power "n"	Logarithm$_{10}$
1000	10^3	3.0
100	10^2	2.0
10	10^1	1.0
1	10^0	0
0.1	10^{-1}	−1.0
0.01	10^{-2}	−2.0
0.0000001	10^{-7}	−7.0.

Figure 1.2 Examples of numbers and their logarithms.

Number	Logarithm$_{10}$
1	0
2	0.301
3	0.477
4	0.602
5	0.699
6	0.778
7	0.845
8	0.903
9	0.954
10	1.0
20	1.301
30	1.477
200	2.301
2000	3.301

Units	Alternative representations	
1 Mole per litre	1 Mol/litre	1 M
0.001 Mole per litre	1 milliMol/litre	1 mM
0.000 001 Mole per litre	1 microMol/litre	1 μM
0.000 000 001 Mole per litre	1 nanoMol/litre	1 nM

Figure 1.3 Understanding units.

pH value	Equivalent in other concentration units
pH 1	0.1 Moles hydrogen ions/litre, or
	10^{-1} Moles hydrogen ions/litre, or
	10^{-1} g hydrogen ions per litre
pH 14	0.000 000 000 000 01 Moles/litre, or
	10^{-14} Moles hydrogen ions/litre, or
	10^{-14} g hydrogen ions /litre

Figure 1.5 pH and equivalent values.

Definition of a base:
A base is a substance which accepts a proton (i.e. a hydrogen ion, H^+) to form an acid. e.g. lactate is a conjugate base which accepts a proton to form lactic acid.
Definition of an acid:
An acid is a compound which dissociates in water to release a proton (ie a hydrogen ion, H^+) e.g. lactic acid
A strong acid
(e.g. hydrochloric acid) is one which readily dissociates in water to release a proton.
A weak acid
(e.g. uric acid) is one which does not readily dissociate in water (e.g. to form urate and a proton).

Figure 1.4 Bronsted and Lowry definition of acids and bases.

Acidotic arterial blood pH values		Clinical examples
pH 6.8	160 nMoles/litre	
pH 6.9	130 nMoles/litre	metabolic acidosis eg diabetic ketoacidosis, renal tubular acidosis
pH 7.0	100 nMoles /litre	
pH 7.1	80 nMoles /litre	
pH 7.2	63 nMoles /litre	respiratory acidosis
pH 7.3	50 nMoles./litre	
Normal arterial blood pH values		
pH 7.35	45 nMoles /litre	
pH 7.36	44 nMoles /litre	normal arterial blood pH
pH 7.38	42 nMoles /litre	
pH 7.40	40 nMoles /litre	pH range is 7.35 to 7.45 (45 to 35 nMoles H$^+$/litre)
pH 7.42	38 nMoles /litre	
pH 7.44	36 nMoles /litre	
pH 7.45	35 nMoles /litre	
Alkalotic arterial blood pH values		**Clinical examples**
pH 7.5	32 nMoles /litre	
pH 7.6	26 nMoles./litre	
pH 7.7	20 nMoles /litre	metabolic alkalosis
pH 7.8	16 nMoles /litre	respiratory alkalosis
pH 7.9	13 nMoles /litre	
pH 8.0	10 nMoles /litre	

Figure 1.6 Examples of pH values seen in clinical practice.

What is pH?

pH is "the "**p**ower of **H**ydrogen". It represents "the negative logarithm$_{10}$ of the hydrogen ion concentration". So why make things so complicated: why not use the plain and simple "hydrogen ion concentration?" Well, the concept was invented by a chemist for chemists and has advantages in chemistry laboratories. In clinical practice we are concerned with arterial values between pH 6.9 and 7.9. However, chemists need to span the entire range of pH values from pH 1 to pH 14. Values in terms of pH enable a convenient compression of numbers compared with the alternative which would be extremely wide-ranging as shown in Fig. 1.3. Figure 1.6 shows the normal reference range for pH in blood and, *in extremis*, fatal ranges which may be seen in acidotic or alkalotic diseases.

The pH scale is not linear:

"The patient's blood pH has changed by 0.3 pH unit" means it has doubled (or halved) in value.

It is sometimes stated that "The patient's arterial blood pH has increased/decreased by, for example, 0.2 pH unit". However, notice that because of the logarithmic scale, this can misrepresent the true change in traditional concentration units. For example, a fall of 0.2 pH units from pH 7.20 to pH 7.00 represents 37 nMol/L, whereas a decrease from pH 7.00 to pH 6.8 represents a change of 60 nMol/L.

However, note that because the $\log_{10}$ of 2 = 0.3 (that is $2 = 10^{0.3}$), a decrease in pH by 0.3, e.g. from pH 7.40 to pH 7.10, represents a two-fold increase in H$^+$ concentration, i.e. from 40 nMol/L to 80 nMol/L.

Similarly, an increase in pH from pH 7.40 to pH 7.70 represents a fall in H$^+$ concentration from 40 nMol/L to 20 nMol/L.

The Henderson-Hasselbalch equation

A weak acid dissociates as shown

$$HB \rightleftharpoons H^+ + B^-$$

weak acid   proton + conjugate base

where **HB is the weak acid** which dissociates to a proton **H$^+$** and its **conjugate base B$^-$** (*NB traditionally authors refer to the conjugate Base as "A$^-$", i.e. the initial letter of Acid which is perhaps confusing*).

Therefore from the Law of Mass Action where K = dissociation constant:

$$K = \frac{[H^+]+[B^-]}{[HB]}$$

Taking logs:

$$\log K = \log[H^+] + \log[B^-] - \log[HB]$$
$$\therefore \ -\log[H^+] = -\log K + \log[B^-] - \log[HB]$$
$$\text{i.e. } pH = pK + \log\frac{[B^-]}{[HB]}$$

Hence the Henderson-Hasselbalch equation:

$$pH = pK + \log\frac{[\text{conjugate base}]}{[\text{acid}]}$$

Clinical relevance of the Henderson-Hasselbalch equation

This is illustrated by respiratory acidosis and respiratory alkalosis.
The equation shows that:

$$pH = pK + \log\frac{[\text{conjugate base}]}{[\text{acid}]}$$

Therefore in the case of the bicarbonate buffer system:

$$pH \propto \log\frac{[HCO_3^-]}{pCO_2}$$

Or alternatively, the hydrogen ion concentration $[H^+] \propto \dfrac{pCO_2}{[HCO_3^-]}$

In other words, the hydrogen ion concentration is proportional to the ratio of the amount of CO_2 to bicarbonate concentration in the blood. Hence, in **hypercapnia** (high blood CO_2 concentration) such as in respiratory acidosis, the ratio of pCO_2 to HCO_3^- is abnormally **high**, therefore the [H$^+$] is **high** (i.e. pH is **low**).

Alternatively, **hypocapnia** caused by hyperventilation results in respiratory alkalosis. In this condition, **low** blood CO_2 concentrations prevail so the hydrogen ion concentration [H$^+$] is **low** (i.e. pH is **high**).

The clinical relevance of pH and buffers will be described further in Chapters 2–5.

2 Understanding pH

Why do so many students have difficulty understanding acid/base theory?
The arcane jargon used in acid-base theory bewilders

Acid/base theory is often considered a difficult subject. It involves an understanding of acids and their ability to dissociate to form a conjugate base and hydrogen ions H^+ (which are "protons"). As long ago as 1962 Creese *et al* wrote in *The Lancet**: **"There is a bewildering variety of** *pseudoscientific jargon in medical writing on this subject"*. Difficulties arise because of this antiquated nomenclature, which is illustrated by the following dialogue:

*Creese R , Neil MW, Ledingham JM, Vere DW (1962) The terminology of acid-base regulation *The Lancet i*, 419.

Student

The patient in intensive care with **lactic acidosis** pH 7.15, has an arterial blood **lactate** of 5.4 mMol/litre. What's the difference between lactic acid and lactate?

Student

Oh, so if the lactic acid is almost completely dissociated does that mean there is very little **lactic acid** present in blood in lactic acidosis?

Professor

Lactic **acid** almost completely dissociates at normal blood pH to form its conjugate base **lactate** and a **proton** (H^+). (Professor scribbles the structures on the back of an envelope):

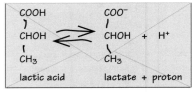

lactic acid   lactate + proton

Professor

Well, yes. At pH 7.15 I calculate from the Henderson-Hasselbalch equation that there are 2000 molecules of lactate for each molecule of lactic acid, (see the Professor's calculation below.)

$$pH = pK + \log \frac{[B^-]}{[HB]}$$ At pH 7.15, given the pK for lactic acid is 3.85 then $$7.15 = 3.85 + \log \frac{lactate}{lactic\ acid}$$

$$\log \frac{lactate}{lactic\ acid} = 7.15 - 3.85 = 3.30$$ Therefore taking antilogs, $$\frac{lactate}{lactic\ acid} = 2000$$

This means that at pH 7.15, there are 2000 molecules of lactate for each molecule of lactic acid, or the proportion of lactic acid is a trivial 0.05%

Student

Well, so is it the supranormal concentration of the conjugate *base* **lactate** which is present in the blood?

Professor

Well, yes

Student

And is it this supranormal concentration of the lactate which is potentially fatal?

Professor

No. In fact, lactate is a "**good**" molecule It's a useful metabolic precursor for gluconeogenesis. It is the supranormal concentration of **protons** which is harmful.

Student

Oh, I see......and the **higher** the concentration of protons, the **lower** the pH.

Professor

Exactly, since pH is the negative logarithm to the base 10 of the hydrogen ion (ie proton) concentration

Professor

Student

(sensing victory) So, this means that when we say the arterial blood is **acidic**, paradoxically there is **very little acid present** .....Therefore, wouldn't it be better to call this a "hyper**protonic**" solution?

Professor

Hmmm, well.... Err.

Student

Therefore, in so-called "lactic acidosis" we have excess of the conjugate *base* **lactate** and of **protons** generated by the dissociation, i.e. **absence**, of lactic acid. .... Wouldn't it be more accurate to call this condition, "**lactate hyperprotonaemia ?**".

Professor

Well, I suppose so but it will never catch on!

Dissociation of lactic acid

Figure 2.1 shows how the ratio of lactate/lactic acid varies with pH. When the proportion of lactate and lactic acid are identical (ie the ratio is 1), the pH equals the pK for lactic acid i.e. the pK for lactic acid is 3.85.

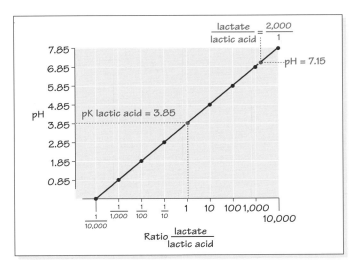

Figure 2.1 The relationship between the dissociation of lactic acid and pH., showing how the ratio of lactate/lactic acid varies with pH. When the proportion of lactate and lactic acid are identical (i.e. the ratio is 1), the pH equals the pK for lactic acid (i.e. the pK of lactic acid is 3.85).

Lactic acid and the bicarbonate buffer system

It takes only a few minutes to demonstrate this at home *in vivo*. Simply exercise anaerobically by running as fast as you can, preferably uphill, until you are breathless. In this time through anaerobic glycolysis, your muscles will have generated **lactic acid** which dissociates to **lactate** and a **proton [H$^+$]** (Fig. 2.2)‡. The protons must be removed and this is achieved when **bicarbonate** reacts with **[H$^+$]** to form **carbonic acid** which spontaneously breaks down to water and CO$_2$. The increased concentration of CO$_2$ stimulates the lungs to hyperventilate thereby blowing off the excess CO$_2$ formed.

‡ The production of protons accompanying the formation of lactate shown in Fig. 2.2 is not strictly correct and has been fudged just as it has been in (probably) all textbooks. Readers who are not satisfied with this traditional (but incorrect) explanation of proton production should read: Robergs RA, Ghiasvand F, Parker D, (2004) Biochemistry of exercise-induced metabolic acidosis *Am J Physiol Regul Integr Comp Physiol* **287**, R502–R516.

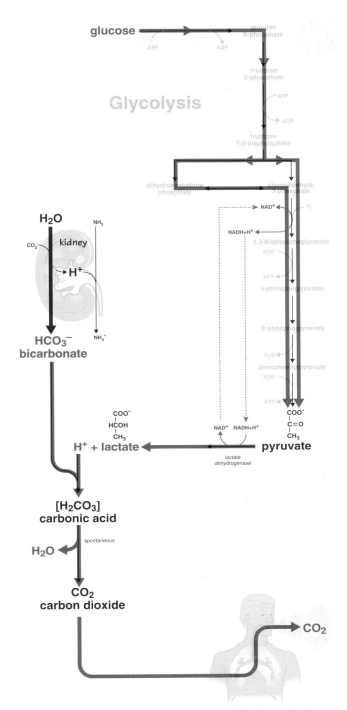

Figure 2.2 Lactic acid and pH homeostasis by the bicarbonate buffer system. The bicarbonate buffer system removes protons [H$^+$] generated during anaerobic glycolysis. The protons are disposed of as water while the CO$_2$ evolved is expired via the lungs.

Production and removal of protons into and from the blood

Protons are produced by metabolism
1. From carbon dioxide
Tissue metabolism of glucose, fatty acids and amino acids generates CO_2 which reacts with water in the presence of **carbonic anhydrase** to form carbonic acid which dissociates to produce bicarbonate and a proton. **This reaction means that carbon dioxide can be thought of as a weak acid.**

$$CO_2 + H_2O \xrightarrow{\text{carbonic anhydrase}} H_2CO_3 \longrightarrow HCO_3^- + H^+$$

carbon + water   carbonic   bicarbonate + proton
dioxide   acid

2. Anaerobic glucose metabolism, ketogenesis, and catabolism of methionine and cysteine produce protons.
(i) The process of anaerobic glycolysis to form lactate produces protons (Chapter 22).

$$\text{glucose} \longrightarrow \text{lactate}^- + H^+$$

(ii) Similarly, protons are formed during the production of acetoacetate and β-hydroxybutryate from fatty acids (Chapter 31).

(iii) **methionine** $\longrightarrow H_2SO_4 \longrightarrow SO_4^{2-} + 2H^+$

(iv) **cysteine** $\longrightarrow H_2SO_4 \longrightarrow SO_4^{2-} + 2H^+$

Kidney glomerulus

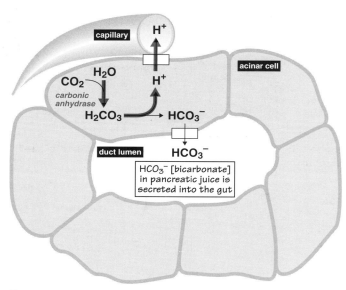

Figure 3.1 Secretion of protons into the blood by the acinar cell of the pancreas.

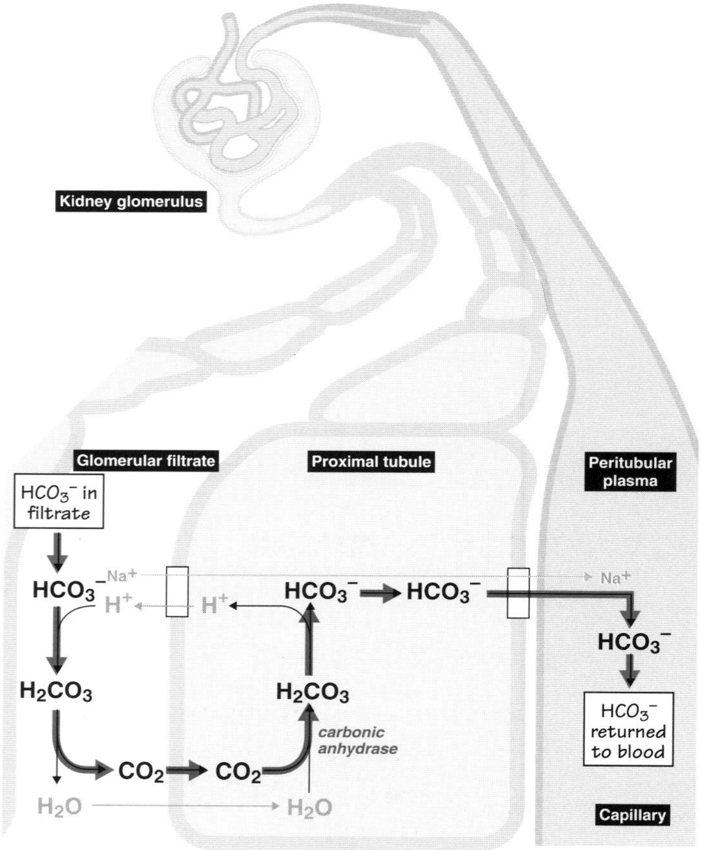

Figure 3.2 Reabsorption of bicarbonate from the renal glomerular filtrate into the blood.

The pancreas secretes protons into the blood.
The acinar cells surrounding the pancreatic duct produce pancreatic juice. This contains a high concentration (up to 125 mMol/l) of HCO_3^- ions which when secreted into the gut neutralises the acidic products from the stomach. The secretion of HCO_3^- into the pancreatic juice is accompanied by an equivalent secretion of protons into the blood, Figure 3.1

The role of the kidney in regulating blood proton concentration.
The kidney plays a major role in regulating plasma pH. It (i) removes protons into the urine and (ii) regulates the concentration of plasma HCO_3^-.
Bicarbonate reabsorption.
Figure 3.2 shows how HCO_3^- is reabsorbed from the glomerular filtrate into the blood.

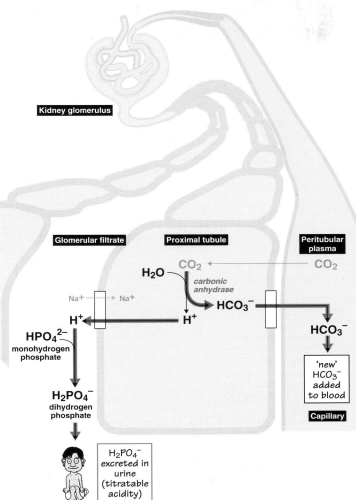

Figure 3.4 Production of "new" bicarbonate linked to excretion of dihydrogen phosphate ions.

> **Production of "new" bicarbonate is linked to excretion of protons in the urine.**
>
> Apart from reabsorbing filtered HCO_3^-, the kidney can also make "new" bicarbonate. This process is associated with either:
>
> **(i) the excretion of protons combined with NH_3 to form NH_4^+ (Fig 3.3).**
>
> The carbonic anhydrase reaction forms protons (H^+) and the "new HCO_3^-" is secreted into the peritubular plasma. The protons must now be excreted by a process involving glutamine. Glutamine is produced by muscle and is deaminated by glutaminase to glutamate which in turn is deaminated by glutamate dehydrogenase. In both cases ammonia NH_3 is formed which diffuses into the glomerular filtrate. Here the NH_3 associates with H^+ forming NH_4^+ which is excreted in the urine.
>
> **(ii) the combination of protons with hydrogen phosphate ions to form dihydrogen phosphate ions (Fig 3.4).**
>
> As in (i) above, the carbonic anhydrase reaction forms protons (H^+) and the "new HCO_3^-" is secreted into the peritubular plasma. This time, the protons (H^+) associate with monohydrogen phosphate ions (HPO_4^{2-}) to form dihydrogen phosphate ($H_2PO_4^-$) which is excreted in the urine.

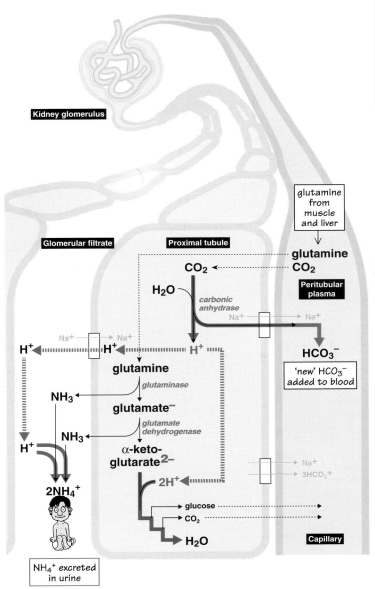

Figure 3.3 Production of "new" bicarbonate linked to excretion of ammonium ions.

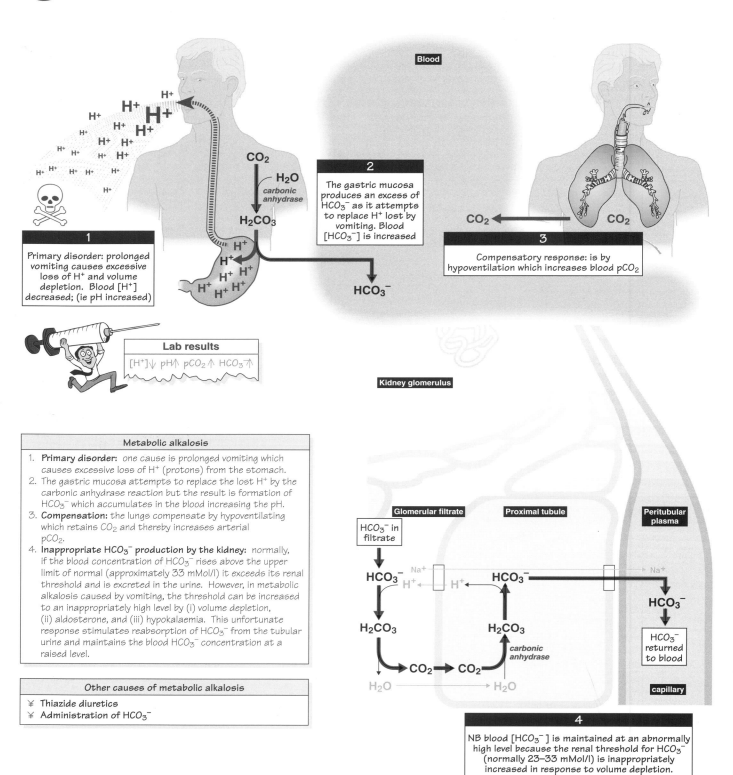

Metabolic alkalosis

1. **Primary disorder:** one cause is prolonged vomiting which causes excessive loss of H+ (protons) from the stomach.
2. The gastric mucosa attempts to replace the lost H+ by the carbonic anhydrase reaction but the result is formation of HCO_3^- which accumulates in the blood increasing the pH.
3. **Compensation:** the lungs compensate by hypoventilating which retains CO_2 and thereby increases arterial pCO_2.
4. **Inappropriate HCO_3^- production by the kidney:** normally, if the blood concentration of HCO_3^- rises above the upper limit of normal (approximately 33 mMol/l) it exceeds its renal threshold and is excreted in the urine. However, in metabolic alkalosis caused by vomiting, the threshold can be increased to an inappropriately high level by (i) volume depletion, (ii) aldosterone, and (iii) hypokalaemia. This unfortunate response stimulates reabsorption of HCO_3^- from the tubular urine and maintains the blood HCO_3^- concentration at a raised level.

Other causes of metabolic alkalosis

¥ Thiazide diuretics
¥ Administration of HCO_3^-

Figure 4.1 Metabolic alkalosis.

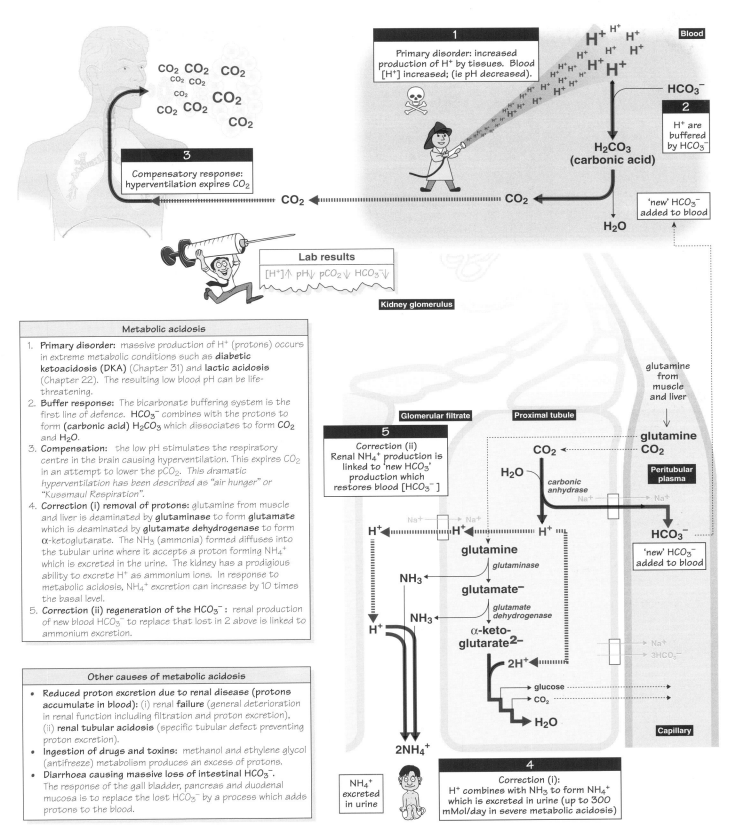

Metabolic acidosis

1. **Primary disorder:** massive production of H^+ (protons) occurs in extreme metabolic conditions such as **diabetic ketoacidosis (DKA)** (Chapter 31) and **lactic acidosis** (Chapter 22). The resulting low blood pH can be life-threatening.

2. **Buffer response:** The bicarbonate buffering system is the first line of defence. HCO_3^- combines with the protons to form (carbonic acid) H_2CO_3 which dissociates to form CO_2 and H_2O.

3. **Compensation:** the low pH stimulates the respiratory centre in the brain causing hyperventilation. This expires CO_2 in an attempt to lower the pCO_2. This dramatic hyperventilation has been described as "air hunger" or "Kussmaul Respiration".

4. **Correction (i) removal of protons:** glutamine from muscle and liver is deaminated by **glutaminase** to form **glutamate** which is deaminated by **glutamate dehydrogenase** to form α-ketoglutarate. The NH_3 (ammonia) formed diffuses into the tubular urine where it accepts a proton forming NH_4^+ which is excreted in the urine. The kidney has a prodigious ability to excrete H^+ as ammonium ions. In response to metabolic acidosis, NH_4^+ excretion can increase by 10 times the basal level.

5. **Correction (ii) regeneration of the HCO_3^-:** renal production of new blood HCO_3^- to replace that lost in 2 above is linked to ammonium excretion.

Other causes of metabolic acidosis

- **Reduced proton excretion due to renal disease (protons accumulate in blood):** (i) renal **failure** (general deterioration in renal function including filtration and proton excretion), (ii) **renal tubular acidosis** (specific tubular defect preventing proton excretion).
- **Ingestion of drugs and toxins:** methanol and ethylene glycol (antifreeze) metabolism produces an excess of protons.
- **Diarrhoea causing massive loss of intestinal HCO_3^-.** The response of the gall bladder, pancreas and duodenal mucosa is to replace the lost HCO_3^- by a process which adds protons to the blood.

Figure 4.2 Metabolic acidosis.

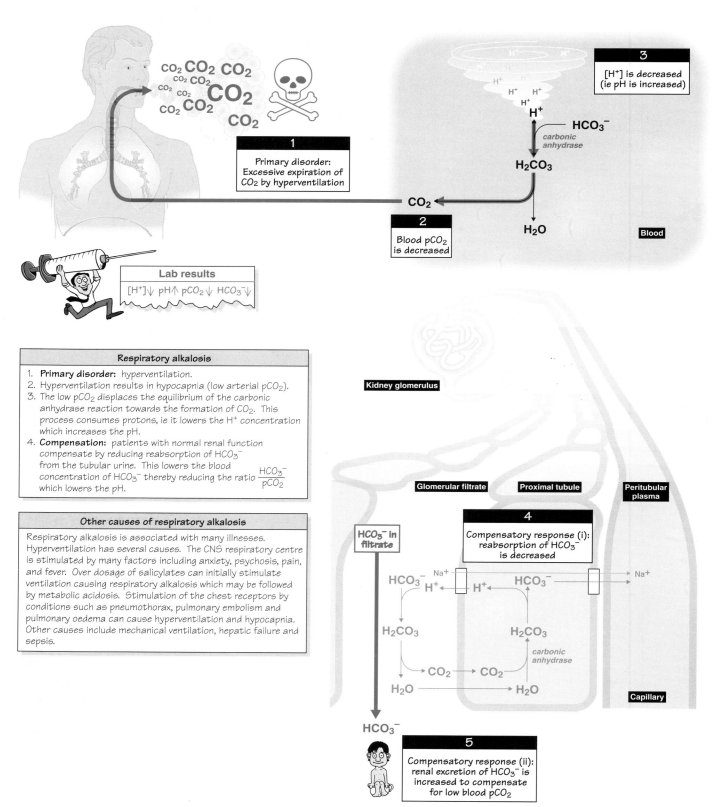

Primary disorder:
Excessive expiration of CO_2 by hyperventilation

1

2
Blood pCO_2
is decreased

3
$[H^+]$ is decreased
(ie pH is increased)

carbonic
anhydrase

Blood

Lab results
$[H^+]\downarrow$ pH$\uparrow$ $pCO_2\downarrow$ $HCO_3^-\downarrow$

Respiratory alkalosis

1. **Primary disorder:** hyperventilation.
2. Hyperventilation results in hypocapnia (low arterial pCO_2).
3. The low pCO_2 displaces the equilibrium of the carbonic anhydrase reaction towards the formation of CO_2. This process consumes protons, ie it lowers the H^+ concentration which increases the pH.
4. **Compensation:** patients with normal renal function compensate by reducing reabsorption of HCO_3^- from the tubular urine. This lowers the blood concentration of HCO_3^- thereby reducing the ratio $\dfrac{HCO_3^-}{pCO_2}$ which lowers the pH.

Other causes of respiratory alkalosis

Respiratory alkalosis is associated with many illnesses. Hyperventilation has several causes. The CNS respiratory centre is stimulated by many factors including anxiety, psychosis, pain, and fever. Over dosage of salicylates can initially stimulate ventilation causing respiratory alkalosis which may be followed by metabolic acidosis. Stimulation of the chest receptors by conditions such as pneumothorax, pulmonary embolism and pulmonary oedema can cause hyperventilation and hypocapnia. Other causes include mechanical ventilation, hepatic failure and sepsis.

Kidney glomerulus

Glomerular filtrate   **Proximal tubule**   **Peritubular plasma**

HCO_3^- in
filtrate

4
Compensatory response (i):
reabsorption of HCO_3^-
is decreased

carbonic
anhydrase

Capillary

HCO_3^-

5
Compensatory response (ii):
renal excretion of HCO_3^- is
increased to compensate
for low blood pCO_2

Figure 5.1 Respiratory alkalosis

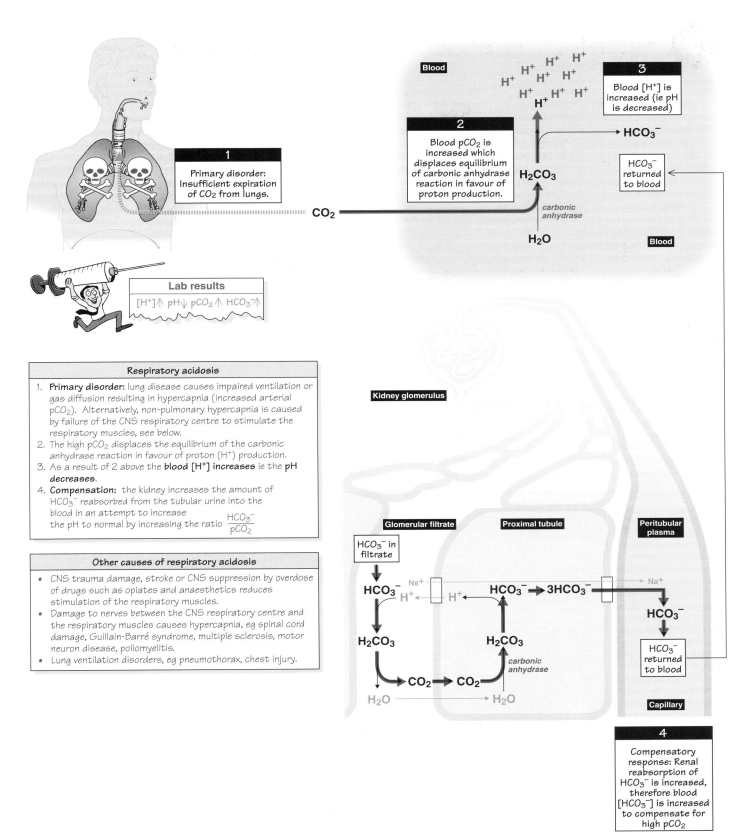

1

Primary disorder: Insufficient expiration of CO_2 from lungs.

Blood

H^+ H^+ H^+ H^+ H^+ H^+ H^+ H^+ H^+ H^+ H^+ H^+ H^+

H^+

2

Blood pCO_2 is increased which displaces equilibrium of carbonic anhydrase reaction in favour of proton production.

3

Blood $[H^+]$ is increased (ie pH is decreased)

HCO_3^-

H_2CO_3

carbonic anhydrase

H_2O

Blood

CO_2

HCO_3^- returned to blood

Lab results

$[H^+] \uparrow$ $pH \downarrow$ $pCO_2 \uparrow$ $HCO_3^- \uparrow$

Respiratory acidosis

1. **Primary disorder:** lung disease causes impaired ventilation or gas diffusion resulting in hypercapnia (increased arterial pCO_2). Alternatively, non-pulmonary hypercapnia is caused by failure of the CNS respiratory centre to stimulate the respiratory muscles, see below.
2. The high pCO_2 displaces the equilibrium of the carbonic anhydrase reaction in favour of proton (H^+) production.
3. As a result of 2 above the **blood $[H^+]$ increases** ie the **pH decreases**.
4. **Compensation:** the kidney increases the amount of HCO_3^- reabsorbed from the tubular urine into the blood in an attempt to increase the pH to normal by increasing the ratio $\dfrac{HCO_3^-}{pCO_2}$

Other causes of respiratory acidosis

- CNS trauma damage, stroke or CNS suppression by overdose of drugs such as opiates and anaesthetics reduces stimulation of the respiratory muscles.
- Damage to nerves between the CNS respiratory centre and the respiratory muscles causes hypercapnia, eg spinal cord damage, Guillain-Barré syndrome, multiple sclerosis, motor neuron disease, poliomyelitis.
- Lung ventilation disorders, eg pneumothorax, chest injury.

Kidney glomerulus

Glomerular filtrate

HCO_3^- in filtrate

HCO_3^-

H_2CO_3

CO_2

H_2O

Proximal tubule

Na^+

H^+ H^+

CO_2

carbonic anhydrase

H_2O

HCO_3^- → $3HCO_3^-$

H_2CO_3

Peritubular plasma

Na^+

HCO_3^-

HCO_3^- returned to blood

Capillary

4

Compensatory response: Renal reabsorption of HCO_3^- is increased, therefore blood $[HCO_3^-]$ is increased to compensate for high pCO_2

Figure 5.2 Respiratory acidosis

6 Amino acids and the primary structure of proteins

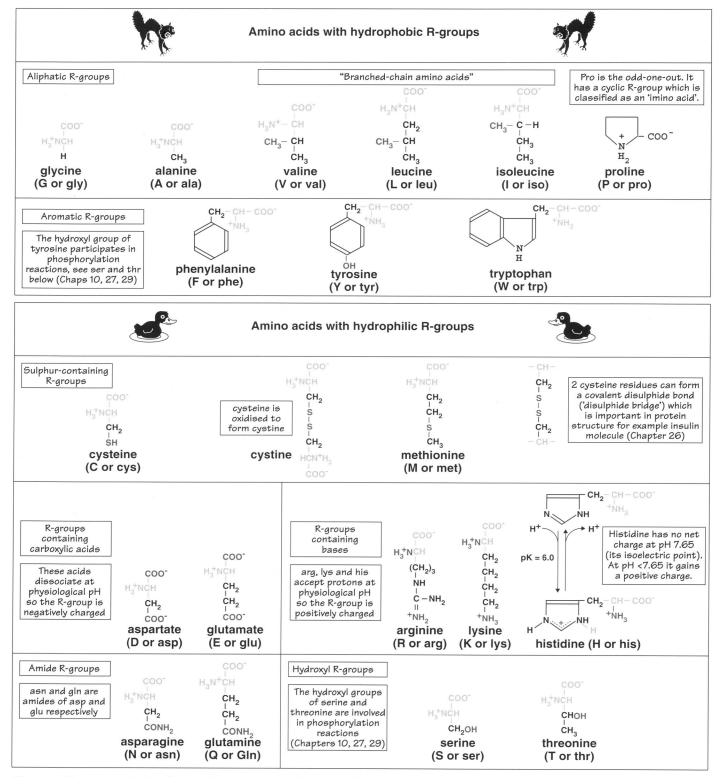

Amino acids with hydrophobic R-groups

Aliphatic R-groups

"Branched-chain amino acids"

Pro is the odd-one-out. It has a cyclic R-group which is classified as an 'imino acid'.

glycine (G or gly)

alanine (A or ala)

valine (V or val)

leucine (L or leu)

isoleucine (I or iso)

proline (P or pro)

Aromatic R-groups

The hydroxyl group of tyrosine participates in phosphorylation reactions, see ser and thr below (Chaps 10, 27, 29)

phenylalanine (F or phe)

tyrosine (Y or tyr)

tryptophan (W or trp)

Amino acids with hydrophilic R-groups

Sulphur-containing R-groups

cysteine is oxidised to form cystine

2 cysteine residues can form a covalent disulphide bond ('disulphide bridge') which is important in protein structure for example insulin molecule (Chapter 26)

cysteine (C or cys)

cystine

methionine (M or met)

R-groups containing carboxylic acids

These acids dissociate at physiological pH so the R-group is negatively charged

aspartate (D or asp)

glutamate (E or glu)

R-groups containing bases

arg, lys and his accept protons at physiological pH so the R-group is positively charged

pK = 6.0

Histidine has no net charge at pH 7.65 (its isoelectric point). At pH <7.65 it gains a positive charge.

arginine (R or arg)

lysine (K or lys)

histidine (H or his)

Amide R-groups

asn and gln are amides of asp and glu respectively

asparagine (N or asn)

glutamine (Q or Gln)

Hydroxyl R-groups

The hydroxyl groups of serine and threonine are involved in phosphorylation reactions (Chapters 10, 27, 29)

serine (S or ser)

threonine (T or thr)

Figure 6.1 The amino acids classified according to their solubility in water. The R group, which is either hydrophilic or hydrophobic, determines their solubility.

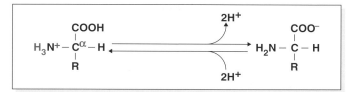

Figure 6.2 General structure of an amino acid.

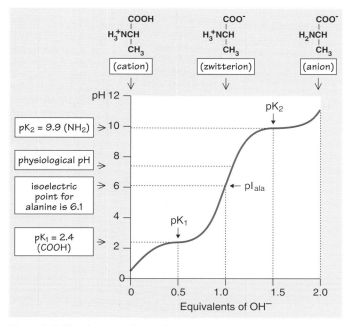

Figure 6.3 Titration curve for alanine.

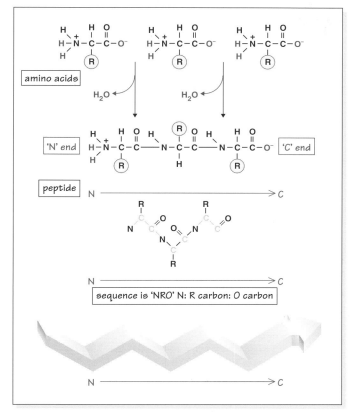

Figure 6.4 Primary structure of a protein. Polymerisation of amino acids to form a polypeptide chain. This is represented as a zig-zag with an arrow head at the C-terminus.

Amino acids

There are 20 amino acids which are the building blocks of proteins (Fig. 6.1). Amino acids are joined by peptide bonds in a precise order which determines the **primary structure** of a protein.

Amino acids have an α-**carbon atom** with bonds to: an **amino** group, a **carboxylic acid** group, a **hydrogen atom** and an "**R" group** which is specific for each amino acid (Fig. 6.2). At physiological pH 7.4, the carboxylic acid dissociates to liberate a proton (**H⁺**) and form a carboxyl group (**COO⁻**), while the amino group accepts a proton (H⁺) to form (**NH₃⁺**). Thus at pH 7.4 an amino acid can have both a positive and a negative charge and is known as a **zwitterion** (from German meaning hybrid ion). The dissociation of **alanine** is shown in its titration curve (Fig. 6.3).

At **low pH** (**i.e. high H⁺** concentration) the carboxyl and amino groups of alanine both **gain** a **H⁺**, giving the **cation** form (i.e. **neutral COOH** and **positively charged NH₃⁺**).

Mnemonic: ca†*ion has a* † *(positive) charge.*

At **high pH** (i.e. low H⁺ concentration) the carboxyl and amino groups both **lose** a **H⁺**, giving the **anion** form (**negative COO⁻** and **neutral NH₂**.

Primary structure

Proteins are a specific sequence of amino acids arranged in a **polypeptide chain** that has an **N terminus** (**H₃N⁺**), and a **C terminus** (**COO⁻**) (Fig. 6.4). The amino acid sequence defines the **primary structure** and determines how the protein folds into its three dimensional shape.

7 Secondary structure of proteins

Secondary structure

Secondary structure largely depends on hydrogen bonding involving the peptide bonds, whereas tertiary structure (Chapter 8) depends on bonds involving the R-groups.

β-strands and β-sheets

The polypeptide chain is organised as β-**strands**. When several of these β-strands associate they form parallel or anti-parallel β-**sheets** (Figs 7.1 and 7.2).

α-helices

Polypeptide chains associate by hydrogen bonds to form a **right-handed α-helix** (Fig. 7.3 opposite).

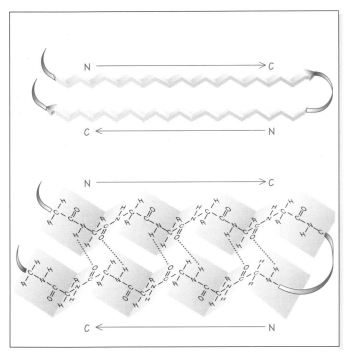

Figure 7.1 Anti-parallel β-sheet. The polypeptide chains organise in a zig-zag manner to form β-strands. The β-strands can associate by hydrogen bonding to form a β-sheet. When two strands run in opposite directions, they are described as "anti-parallel".

Abnormal primary structure affects the secondary structure: deletion of a single amino acid causes cystic fibrosis

The primary structure refers to the **amino acid sequence of the polypeptide chain**. An error caused by a single incorrect amino acid amongst a chain of 1480 amino acids can seriously affect the function of the protein. This happens in people with **cystic fibrosis** who have a defective **CFTR gene** (**cystic fibrosis transmembrane conductance regulator**) which produces a defective chloride transporter protein.

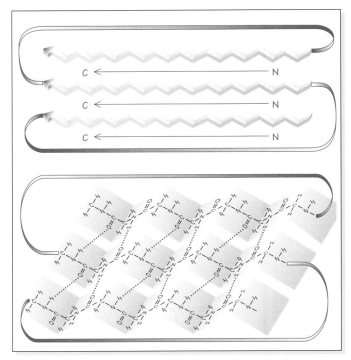

Figure 7.2 Parallel β-sheet. The three β-strands associate by hydrogen bonding to form a β-pleated sheet. The strands run in the same direction and so are described as being "parallel".

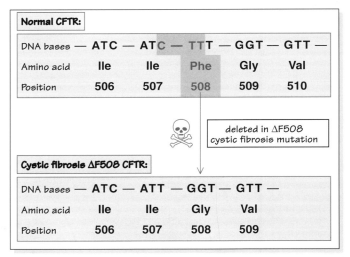

Normal CFTR:

DNA bases —	ATC —	ATC —	TTT —	GGT —	GTT —
Amino acid	Ile	Ile	Phe	Gly	Val
Position	506	507	508	509	510

deleted in ΔF508 cystic fibrosis mutation

Cystic fibrosis ΔF508 CFTR:

DNA bases —	ATC —	ATT —	GGT —	GTT —
Amino acid	Ile	Ile	Gly	Val
Position	506	507	508	509

Figure 7.4 The ΔF508 mutation causes cystic fibrosis. Deletion of bases **CTT** as shown results in loss of **phenylalanine** at position 508 from **the cystic fibrosis transmembrane conductance regulator protein (CFTR)** forming the dysfunctional product which causes cystic fibrosis. NB Isoleucine at 507 is not affected as both **ATC** and **ATT** code for isoleucine.

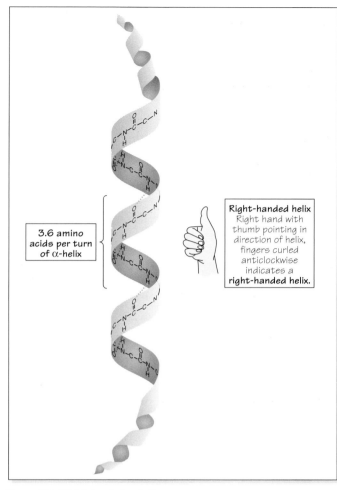

Figure 7.3 Right-handed α-helix.

3.6 amino acids per turn of α-helix

Right-handed helix
Right hand with thumb pointing in direction of helix, fingers curled anticlockwise indicates a right-handed helix.

In 70% of people with cystic fibrosis, the mutation is deletion of three base pairs in the DNA which results in the loss of phenylalanine at position 508 (Fig. 7.4). This is known as the **ΔF508 mutation** (Δ for **deletion**; **F** for **phenylalanine**; **508** for the **position** of this phenylalanine in the primary structure). Following synthesis the abnormal CFTR protein folds into an incorrect **secondary structure** and is retained in the endoplasmic reticulum. Loss of the chloride transporter results in the accumulation of thick, viscous mucus which adversely affects lung function. It also results in defective exocrine pancreatic secretion resulting in a malabsorption syndrome.

Derangement of the secondary structure of a prion protein causes spongiform encephalopathy (e.g. CJD or "mad cow disease")

Prions are proteinaceous infectious particles consisting only of protein and do not contain DNA or RNA. Derangement of the secondary structure of prions results in the spongiform encephalopathies such a **scrapie** (in sheep) and **bovine spongiform encephalopathy (BSE, "mad cow disease")**. Human diseases are: **Creutzfeld-Jacob disease (CJD)**, **kuru** (from cannibalistic practice of eating human brain and "**variant CJD**". Prion protein (PrP^C) is a normal cellular protein of unknown function which is expressed in neurones. As shown in Fig. 7.5, prion normally consists mainly of α-helices. However the PrP^C protein can be corrupted to the malignant form PrP^{SC} (^{SC} for scrapie) which comprises **mainly β-pleated sheets**. This in turn adversely affects the tertiary structure (see below) causing spongiform encephalopathy. The mechanism of the α-helix metamorphosis to a β-pleated sheet is not understood. The presence of an abnormal PrP^{SC} molecule somehow converts PrP^C molecules to PrP^{SC} molecules in a chain reaction which, like a rotten apple in a barrel, propagates disease throughout the brain.

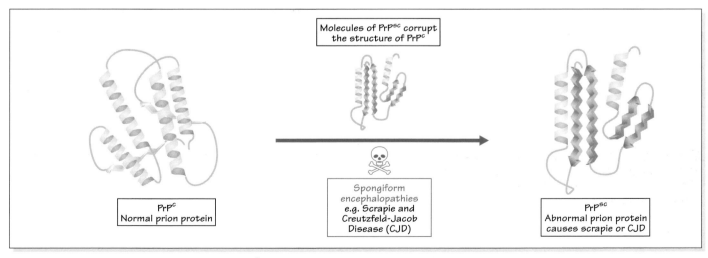

Molecules of PrP^{SC} corrupt the structure of PrP^C

PrP^C
Normal prion protein

Spongiform encephalopathies e.g. Scrapie and Creutzfeld-Jacob Disease (CJD)

PrP^{SC}
Abnormal prion protein causes scrapie or CJD

Figure 7.5 Prion proteins. Normal prion protein (PrP^C) contains a lot of α-helical regions and is soluble. However, in the mutant prion that causes scrapie (PrP^{SC}), some of the α-helix is converted to the β-pleated conformation which is insoluble. The mutant PrP^{SC} is "infectious" because it potentiates the conversion of an α-helix to β-conformation.

8 Tertiary and quaternary structure and collagen

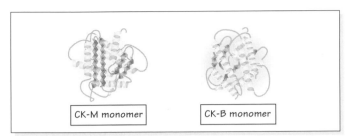

Figure 8.1 Tertiary structure. β-pleated sheets and α-helices fold themselves to form two different **creatine kinase (CK)** monomers (**CK-M** and **CK-B**).

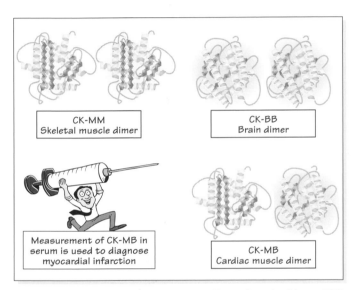

Figure 8.2 Quaternary structure. The two different **Creatine kinase** (CK) monomers (**M** and **B**) associate to form three different dimers: the **homo-**dimers **CK-MM** (found in skeletal muscle) and **CK-BB** (brain), and the **hetero**-dimer **CK-MB** which is abundant in cardiac muscle.

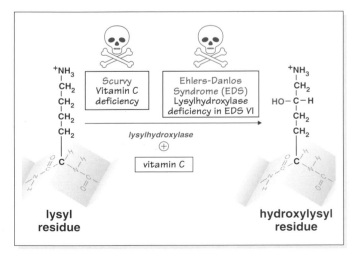

Figure 8.3 Hydroxylation of lysyl residue during collagen formation.

Tertiary structure of protein

When β-**strands**, β-**pleated sheets** and α-**helices** fold together they form the **tertiary** structure of the protein, for example the creatine kinase monomers CK-M and CK-B (Fig. 8.1).

Quaternary structure of protein

Many proteins consist of more than one polypeptide chain which combine by non-covalent forces. The single protein is a **monomer**. Quaternary structure defines the association of monomers to form **dimers** (two monomers) (Fig. 8.2), **trimers** (three), **tetramers** (four), etc. and **oligomers** (composed of many monomers).

Collagen

Currently 19 types of collagen are known (Greek *kola, glue*; produces glue on boiling connective tissue). They are fibrous, structural proteins and are the most abundant protein in humans. Collagens are variably distributed, with type I being mainly found in ligaments, tendons and skin and type II being the principal collagen in cartilage.

Collagen is constructed from α-**chain units** which associate to form a **triple helix**. The primary structure of collagen is repeats of the sequence—**Gly—X—Y**—where **X** is often proline. **Y** is usually a proline residue which has been hydroxylated in a vitamin C-dependent reaction producing a **hydroxyproline** residue. Alternatively, Y can be a **hydroxylysine** residue (Fig. 8.3). **Glycine** (remember its R group is a single hydrogen atom) is an essential component because restricted space in the triple helix does not permit larger molecules.

Biosynthesis of collagen

Collagen is an extracellular, insoluble glycoprotein. This raises the question: how do **fibroblasts**, the collagen-producing cells, make an insoluble extracellular protein? The answer involves an intracellular stage and an extracellular stage (Fig. 8.4).

The intracellular stage produces procollagen

The intracellular protein machinery first of all produces polypeptide α-chains (approximately 1000 amino acids). Some of the prolyl and lysyl residues are hydroxylated by reactions that need vitamin C (Chapter 58). Some of the hydroxylysyl residues are glycosylated. The units then associate to form the triple helix (rope-like) **procollagen** which is soluble.

The extracellular stage produces collagen fibres

Procollagen is secreted from the cell into the extracellular fluid where the terminal globular, **propetides** are removed by **procollagen peptidase**, forming **tropocollagen** which is insoluble. The tropocollagen units assemble into microfibrils in which each collagen unit is staggered so it overlaps its neighbours by one-quarter of the length of a collagen molecule. Finally, **lysyl-oxidase** causes lysyl and hydroxylysyl residues to react forming cross-links which provide tensile strength, and the microfibrils associate to form a polymeric collagen fibre.

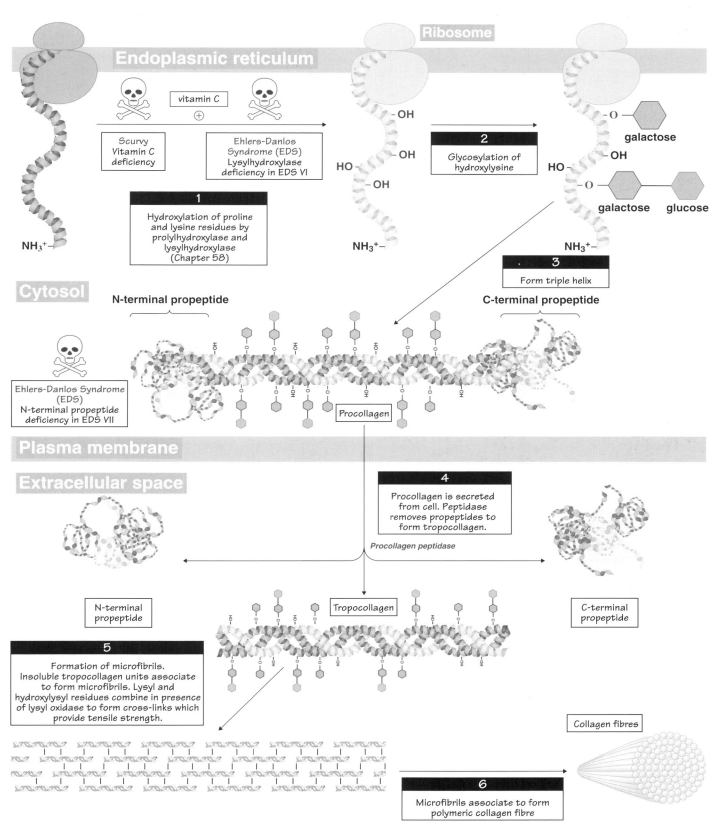

Figure 8.4 Biosynthesis of collagen.

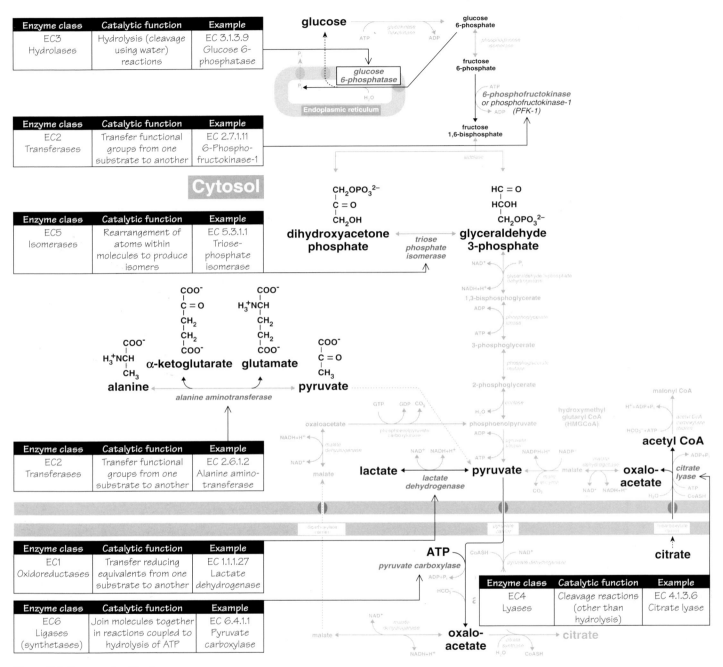

Enzyme class	Catalytic function	Example
EC3 Hydrolases	Hydrolysis (cleavage using water) reactions	EC 3.1.3.9 Glucose 6-phosphatase

Enzyme class	Catalytic function	Example
EC2 Transferases	Transfer functional groups from one substrate to another	EC 2.7.1.11 6-Phospho-fructokinase-1

Enzyme class	Catalytic function	Example
EC5 Isomerases	Rearrangement of atoms within molecules to produce isomers	EC 5.3.1.1 Triose-phosphate isomerase

Enzyme class	Catalytic function	Example
EC2 Transferases	Transfer functional groups from one substrate to another	EC 2.6.1.2 Alanine amino-transferase

Enzyme class	Catalytic function	Example
EC1 Oxidoreductases	Transfer reducing equivalents from one substrate to another	EC 1.1.1.27 Lactate dehydrogenase

Enzyme class	Catalytic function	Example
EC6 Ligases (synthetases)	Join molecules together in reactions coupled to hydrolysis of ATP	EC 6.4.1.1 Pyruvate carboxylase

Enzyme class	Catalytic function	Example
EC4 Lyases	Cleavage reactions (other than hydrolysis)	EC 4.1.3.6 Citrate lyase

Figure 9.1 Enzyme classification.

Enzyme nomenclature

Enzyme nomenclature and classification is according to recommendations of the International Union of Biochemistry and Molecular Biology (**IUBMB**) *www.chem.qmul.ac.uk/iubmb*. Enzymes are classified in **6 classes** (**EC1, EC2, EC3**, etc.) which in turn are divided into subclasses (Fig. 9.1).

Enzyme kinetics: velocity versus substrate concentration curve

Figure 9.2 shows an initial velocity versus substrate concentration curve. The reaction velocity (v) increases in proportion to increasing concentration of substrate [S] until all the catalytic sites of the enzyme are working as fast as they can and maximum reaction velocity (V_{max})

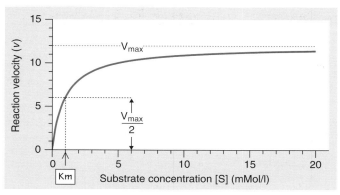

Figure 9.2 Michaelis–Menten plot

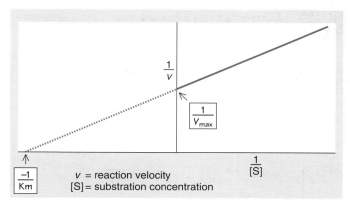

v = reaction velocity
[S] = substration concentration

Figure 9.3 Lineweaver–Burke double reciprocal plot.

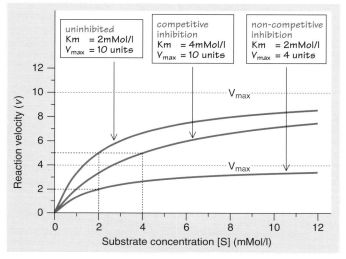

Figure 9.4 Michaelis plot in the presence of competitive and non-competitive inhibitors.

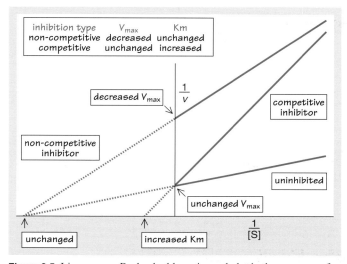

Figure 9.5 Lineweaver–Burke double reciprocal plot in the presence of competitive and non-competitive inhibitors.

(12 units) is approached. From this graph the Michaelis–Menten constant (Km) is obtained. The Km is defined as "the substrate concentration giving half V_{max} ($V_{max}/2$)". In Fig. 9.2 the Km is 1 mMol/l.

If the substrate concentration and reaction velocity are plotted as the reciprocal of their values, a linear relationship is known as the Lineweaver-Burke plot is obtained (Fig. 9.3).

Competitive and non-competitive inhibition

Figure 9.4 shows the Michaelis–Menten v versus [S] plot for an enzyme in the absence and presence of either competitive or non-competitive inhibitors. Figure 9.5 shows the same as a Lineweaver–Burke reciprocal plot. Figure 9.4 shows an uninhibited enzyme which has a V_{max} of 10 units and a Km of 2 mMol/l.

Competitive enzyme inhibitors are used as drugs. They have structures similar to the natural substrate and can therefore compete with it for access to the same binding site on the enzyme. For example **methotrexate** (anticancer drug) structurally resembles **folate,** which is the natural substrate for **dihydrofolate reductase** (Chapter 50). Metho-

trexate is used to inhibit dihydrofolate reductase in cancer chemotherapy.

In Fig. 9.4 we see how an enzyme in the presence of a competitor needs more substrate to beat off the competition. However, given sufficient substrate the competitive inhibitor is overwhelmed, inhibition is reversed, and the enzyme can operate at its normal V_{max}. NB The competitor obstructs the binding site thus **decreasing** the affinity of the enzyme for its substrate, in other words it **increases** the Km e.g. to 4 mMol/l but V_{max} is unchanged.

Non-competitive inhibitors. A non-competitive inhibitor binds to a site other than the substrate binding site therefore inhibition is not overcome by increasing the substrate concentration. In fact, non-competitive inhibition is simply understood by remembering that each substrate has its own sub-binding site. Therefore, increasing the concentration of one substrate will not alter the binding of an inhibitor which is blocking another sub-binding site. Consequently, non-competitive inhibitors affect a fixed proportion of the enzyme molecules, do not change the Km but decrease V_{max} by a constant percentage.

10 Regulation of enzyme activity

Regulation by availability of cofactors

There is not general agreement in terminology but the following is used here. **A cofactor is a general term for a substance, whether organic or inorganic, that is essential for the enzyme to function.** Thus, all the following are cofactors.

Coenzyme A coenzyme is a soluble, organic molecule which promiscuously associates and dissociates with the various enzymes it partners eg NAD^+ and various dehydrogenases (Chapter 13).

Prosthetic Group A prosthetic group, for example **FAD**, is an organic molecule covalently bound to its partner enzyme throughout the lifetime of the enzyme.

Metal-activated enzymes Some enzymes collaborate with soluble metal ion cofactors for example Mg^{++}. Mg^{++} combines with ATP to provide the substrate for kinase reactions eg hexokinase.

Metalloenzymes These are enzymes to which a metal is bound e.g. alcohol dehydrogenase which is a zinc metalloenzyme. Zinc is bound to the sulphur atom of cysteine which is part of the reactive site.

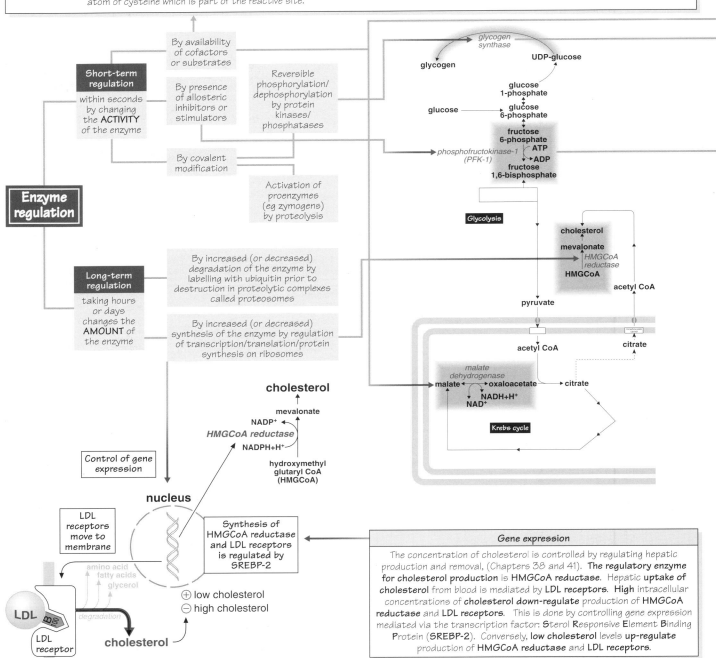

Gene expression

The concentration of cholesterol is controlled by regulating hepatic production and removal, (Chapters 38 and 41). **The regulatory enzyme for cholesterol production is HMGCoA reductase.** Hepatic **uptake of cholesterol** from blood is mediated by **LDL receptors.** High intracellular concentrations of **cholesterol down-regulate** production of **HMGCoA reductase** and **LDL receptors.** This is done by controlling gene expression mediated via the transcription factor: **S**terol **R**esponsive **E**lement **B**inding **P**rotein (**SREBP-2**). Conversely, **low cholesterol** levels **up-regulate** production of **HMGCoA reductase** and **LDL receptors.**

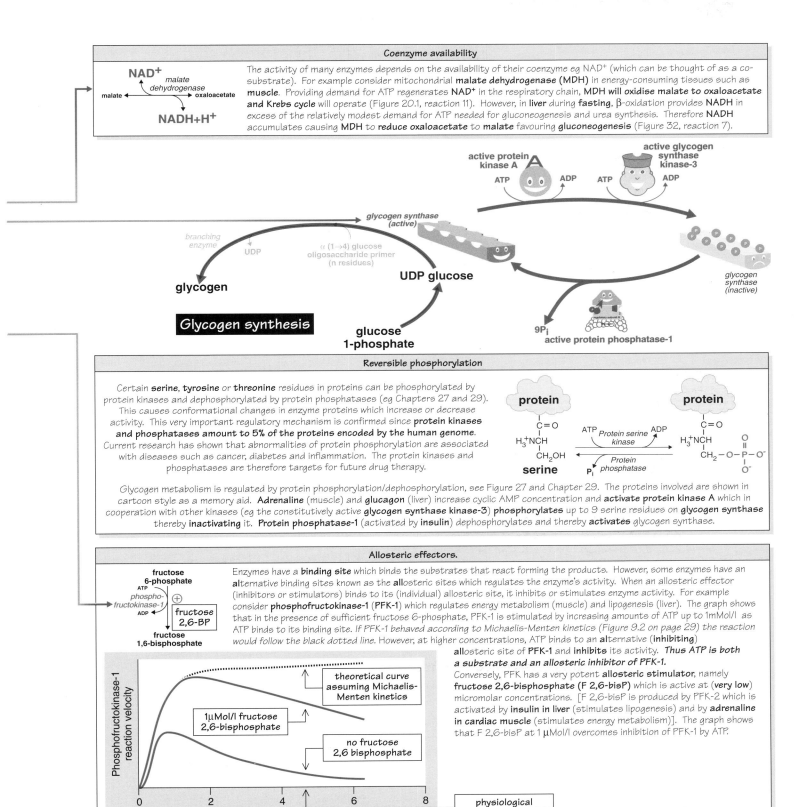

Coenzyme availability

NAD⁺

malate ⇌ oxaloacetate
malate dehydrogenase

NADH+H⁺

The activity of many enzymes depends on the availability of their coenzyme eg NAD⁺ (which can be thought of as a co-substrate). For example consider mitochondrial **malate dehydrogenase (MDH)** in energy-consuming tissues such as **muscle**. Providing demand for ATP regenerates **NAD⁺** in the respiratory chain, **MDH will oxidise malate to oxaloacetate and Krebs cycle** will operate (Figure 20.1, reaction 11). However, in **liver** during **fasting**, β-oxidation provides NADH in excess of the relatively modest demand for ATP needed for gluconeogenesis and urea synthesis. Therefore **NADH** accumulates causing **MDH** to **reduce oxaloacetate** to **malate** favouring **gluconeogenesis** (Figure 32, reaction 7).

active protein kinase A

ATP → ADP

active glycogen synthase kinase-3

ATP → ADP

glycogen synthase (active)

branching enzyme

UDP

α (1→4) glucose oligosaccharide primer (n residues)

UDP glucose

glycogen

Glycogen synthesis

glucose 1-phosphate

glycogen synthase (inactive)

9Pᵢ

active protein phosphatase-1

Reversible phosphorylation

Certain **serine, tyrosine** or **threonine** residues in proteins can be phosphorylated by protein kinases and dephosphorylated by protein phosphatases (eg Chapters 27 and 29). This causes conformational changes in enzyme proteins which increase or decrease activity. This very important regulatory mechanism is confirmed since **protein kinases and phosphatases amount to 5% of the proteins encoded by the human genome**. Current research has shown that abnormalities of protein phosphorylation are associated with diseases such as cancer, diabetes and inflammation. The protein kinases and phosphatases are therefore targets for future drug therapy.

protein

C=O
|
H₃⁺NCH
|
CH₂OH

serine

ATP → ADP
Protein serine kinase

Pᵢ ← *Protein phosphatase*

protein

C=O
|
H₃⁺NCH
|
CH₂−O−P−O⁻

Glycogen metabolism is regulated by protein phosphorylation/dephosphorylation, see Figure 27 and Chapter 29. The proteins involved are shown in cartoon style as a memory aid. **Adrenaline** (muscle) and **glucagon** (liver) increase cyclic AMP concentration and **activate protein kinase A** which in cooperation with other kinases (eg the constitutively active **glycogen synthase kinase-3**) phosphorylates up to 9 serine residues on **glycogen synthase** thereby **inactivating it**. **Protein phosphatase-1** (activated by **insulin**) dephosphorylates and thereby **activates** glycogen synthase.

Allosteric effectors.

fructose 6-phosphate

ATP
phospho-fructokinase-1 ⊕
ADP

fructose 2,6-BP

fructose 1,6-bisphosphate

Enzymes have a **binding site** which binds the substrates that react forming the products. However, some enzymes have an **a**lternative binding sites known as the **allo**steric sites which regulates the enzyme's activity. When an allosteric effector (inhibitors or stimulators) binds to its (individual) allosteric site, it inhibits or stimulates enzyme activity. For example consider **phosphofructokinase-1** (PFK-1) which regulates energy metabolism (muscle) and lipogenesis (liver). The graph shows that in the presence of sufficient fructose 6-phosphate, PFK-1 is stimulated by increasing amounts of ATP up to 1mMol/l as ATP binds to its binding site. If PFK-1 behaved according to Michaelis-Menten kinetics (Figure 9.2 on page 29) the reaction would follow the black dotted line. However, at higher concentrations, ATP binds to an **a**lternative (**inhibiting**) allosteric site of PFK-1 and **inhibits** its activity. **Thus ATP is both a substrate and an allosteric inhibitor of PFK-1.**

Conversely, PFK has a very potent **allosteric stimulator**, namely **fructose 2,6-bisphosphate (F 2,6-bisP)** which is active at (**very low**) micromolar concentrations. [F 2,6-bisP is produced by PFK-2 which is activated by **insulin in liver** (stimulates lipogenesis) and by **adrenaline in cardiac muscle** (stimulates energy metabolism)]. The graph shows that F 2,6-bisP at 1 μMol/l overcomes inhibition of PFK-1 by ATP.

theoretical curve assuming Michaelis-Menten kinetics

1μMol/l fructose 2,6-bisphosphate

no fructose 2,6 bisphosphate

Phosphofructokinase-1 reaction velocity

0   2   4   6   8
ATP concentration (mMol/l)

physiological concentration of ATP

Figure 10.1 Regulation of enzyme activity.

11 Carbohydrates

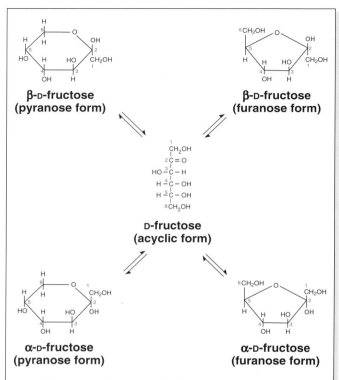

α-D-glucose   **D-glucose (acyclic form)**   **β-D-glucose**

36% α-anomer   **64%** β-anomer

Nomenclature: confusion between D- and L-; d- and l-.

The pioneers of carbohydrate chemistry used the "optical activity" (their ability to rotate the plane of polarised light clockwise or anticlockwise) to characterise carbohydrate structures. They observed that **glucose** and **fructose** rotated light to the **right** and **left** respective and described them as "**d**" (**dextrorotatory**) and "**l**" (**laevorotatory**). (Latin: *dexter* right, and *laevus* left). Later, confusion arose when convention determined that the asymmetric atoms at C5 of **d**- glucose (and inconveniently **l-fructose**!) were configured in the **D**- convention (NB capital D) with the **OH group on the right-hand-side of C5**. Therefore the terms "d" and "l" became obsolete and instead "+" and "-" were introduced to describe optical rotation.

Glucose

The naturally occurring enantiomer of glucose is **D-glucose** also known by the arcane name **dextrose**. In medical circles confusion arises because glucose is often referred to as "dextrose" when it is infused into a patient, while the laboratory reports "**blood glucose**" concentrations. Even in medical literature, both dextrose and glucose are sometimes used in the same paper!

When glucose is dissolved in water, it has a structural identity crisis! It undergoes mutarotation and exists in ring forms or a straight chain. The two ring forms are 36% **α-D-Glucose** or 64% **β-D-glucose** depending on the position of the OH group on the anomeric carbon atom, C1. If the OH group projects downwards, it is the **α-anomer**; if it projects upwards, it is the **β- anomer**. The **acyclic** ("straight chain") intermediate form comprises only 0.003% of the mixture.

Prolonged exposure of body proteins to high concentrations of glucose results in **glycation** which damages the proteins. This is known as "**glucose toxicity**" and is responsible for many of the complications of diabetes mellitus, Chapter 33.

Figure 11.1 Carbohydrate nomenclature.

β-D-fructose (pyranose form)   **β-D-fructose (furanose form)**

D-fructose (acyclic form)

α-D-fructose (pyranose form)   **α-D-fructose (furanose form)**

Naturally occurring **D-fructose** is also known by the arcane name, **laevulose**. Like glucose, fructose in solution also has an identity crisis: it exists in both α- and β- forms which in turn are changing between pyranose rings (6-membered rings) and furanose (5-membered rings). Fructose phosphates exist as furanose rings.

Inulin. Several plants store a polymer of fructose called **inulin** (do not confuse with **insulin**) as a food reserve which is analogous to starch. Onions, leeks and banana contain inulin but it is notoriously present in tubers of Jerusalem artichoke (*Helianthus tuberosus*). Since inulin is poorly digested it causes flatulence hence their irreverent nickname Jerusalem "Fartichokes". On a positive note, the "**inulin clearance test**" is the gold standard test for glomerular filtration since following intravenous infusion it is completely excreted in the urine.

Figure 11.2 Structure of fructose.

Glycogen is a spherical molecule comprising numerous chains of ten glucose molecules α-(1→4) linked which branch at α-(1→6) bonds. It radiates from a central protein, **glycogenin**.

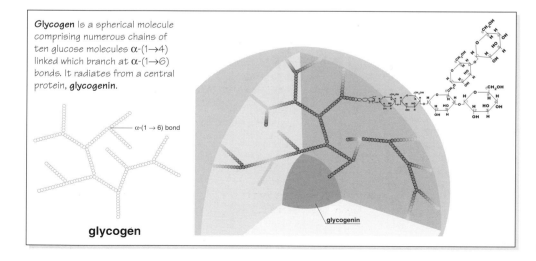

α-(1 → 6) bond

glycogen

glycogenin

Figure 11.3 Glycogen.

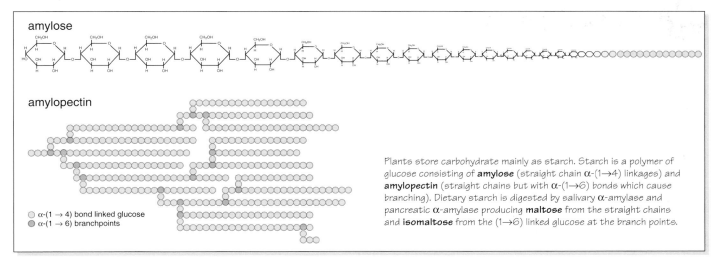

amylose

amylopectin

○ α-(1 → 4) bond linked glucose
● α-(1 → 6) branchpoints

Plants store carbohydrate mainly as starch. Starch is a polymer of glucose consisting of **amylose** (straight chain α-(1→4) linkages) and **amylopectin** (straight chains but with α-(1→6) bonds which cause branching). Dietary starch is digested by salivary α-amylase and pancreatic α-amylase producing **maltose** from the straight chains and **isomaltose** from the (1→6) linked glucose at the branch points.

Figure 11.4 Starch.

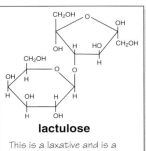

lactulose

This is a laxative and is a synthetic disaccharide comprising galactose and fructose. It is a stool softener, and since it is also a colonic acidifier, it removes ammonia from the blood in liver failure.

Figure 11.5 Lactulose.

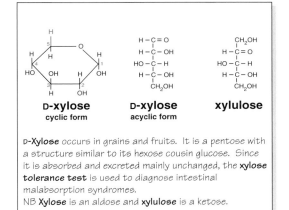

D-xylose
cyclic form

D-xylose
acyclic form

xylulose

D-Xylose occurs in grains and fruits. It is a pentose with a structure similar to its hexose cousin glucose. Since it is absorbed and excreted mainly unchanged, the **xylose tolerance test** is used to diagnose intestinal malabsorption syndromes.
NB **Xylose** is an aldose and **xylulose** is a ketose.

Figure 11.6 D-Xylose and xylulose.

β-D-ribose   **β-2-deoxy-D-ribose**

Ribose is a pentose found in ribonucleic acid (**RNA**).
Deoxyribose, found in deoxyribonucleic acid (**DNA**), is derived from ribose by replacing the hydroxyl group at carbon 2 with hydrogen.

Figure 11.7 Ribose and deoxyribose.

α-D-glucose   α-D-glucose

trehalose

Trehalose occurs in the cocoons of the beetle *Trehala manna* and is thought to be the **manna** of biblical fame. The sweetness of manna is due to **trehalose** (two glucose molecules joined by **α-1 bonding**). Trehalose is found in the haemolymph of insects and in mushrooms. Trehalose **stabilises the tertiary structure of proteins** (Chapter 8) enabling them to resist denaturation when subjected to dehydration. For example, the Resurrection plant or Rose of Jericho (*Selaginella lepidophylla*) which contains trehalose can withstand total drought for several years and when soaked with water will uncurl and flourish. This property of trehalose is used to store proteins such as hormones and antibodies.

Figure 11.8 Trehalose.

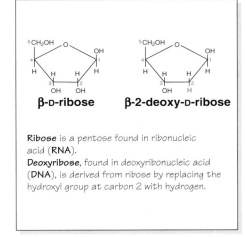

sorbitol   **mannitol**   **galactitol**   **xylitol**

The **sugar alcohols** are polyols.
Sorbitol
Sorbitol was used by diabetic patients as a bulk sweetener. However, it is now considered to be of no benefit.
Intravenous **mannitol** is used as a diuretic.
Galactitol accumulates in people with galactosaemia.
Xylitol is the sugar alcohol form of xylose. It is extracted from birch wood and is also called "wood sugar". Xylitol is used as an anticariogenic sweetener in chewing gum.

Figure 11.9 Sugar alcohols.

12 Absorption of carbohydrates and metabolism of galactose

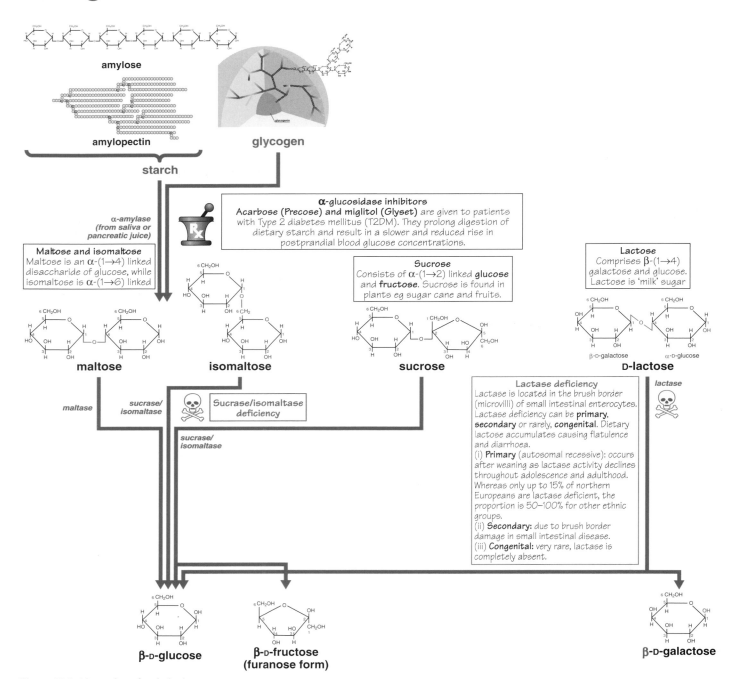

Figure 12.1 Absorption of carbohydrates.

The figure contains the following labels and text boxes:

amylose

amylopectin **glycogen**

starch

α-amylase (from saliva or pancreatic juice)

α-glucosidase inhibitors
Acarbose (Precose) and miglitol (Glyset) are given to patients with Type 2 diabetes mellitus (T2DM). They prolong digestion of dietary starch and result in a slower and reduced rise in postprandial blood glucose concentrations.

Maltose and isomaltose
Maltose is an α-(1→4) linked disaccharide of glucose, while isomaltose is α-(1→6) linked

Sucrose
Consists of α-(1→2) linked **glucose** and **fructose**. Sucrose is found in plants eg sugar cane and fruits.

Lactose
Comprises β-(1→4) galactose and glucose. Lactose is 'milk' sugar

maltose **isomaltose** **sucrose** **D-lactose**

β-D-galactose α-D-glucose

maltase

sucrase/isomaltase

Sucrase/isomaltase deficiency

sucrase/isomaltase

lactase

Lactase deficiency
Lactase is located in the brush border (microvilli) of small intestinal enterocytes. Lactase deficiency can be **primary**, **secondary** or rarely, **congenital**. Dietary lactose accumulates causing flatulence and diarrhoea.
(i) **Primary** (autosomal recessive): occurs after weaning as lactase activity declines throughout adolescence and adulthood. Whereas only up to 15% of northern Europeans are lactase deficient, the proportion is 50–100% for other ethnic groups.
(ii) **Secondary**: due to brush border damage in small intestinal disease.
(iii) **Congenital**: very rare, lactase is completely absent.

β-D-glucose **β-D-fructose (furanose form)** **β-D-galactose**

Galactose metabolism

The main dietary source of galactose is the disaccharide it forms with glucose, namely lactose (Fig. 12.1). **Lactose** (milk sugar) is hydrolysed in the intestine by **lactase** and the **glucose** and **galactose** produced are transported directly to the liver via the hepatic portal vein. Galactose can enter the pathways used for glucose metabolism as follows. It is phosphorylated by **galactokinase** to galactose 1-phosphate. Galactose 1-phosphate in the presence of **gal**actose **1-p**hosphate **u**ridyl**t**ransferase (**Gal 1 PUT**) forms glucose 1-phosphate. Gal 1 Put also forms **UDP galactose** which can also be metabolised to **glucose 1-phosphate** by **epimerase**. The glucose 1-phosphate can be metabolised to glycogen, or to glucose 6-phosphate and then via glycolysis or the pentose phosphate pathway.

Galactose metabolism in disease

Galactose 1-phosphate uridyltransferase deficiency (Gal 1 PUT deficiency) is a rare autosomal recessive disorder which results in galactosaemia and galactosuria. It is usually manifest shortly after birth when the baby has feeding difficulties, with vomiting and failure to thrive. If not treated, liver damage, mental retardation and formation of cataracts can result.

A disease with similar symptoms occurs in **galactokinase** deficiency. In both cases, galactose accumulates and it is reduced to galactitol by aldose reductase.

Treatment is achieved by avoiding galactose and lactose in the diet. (NB Do not confuse these conditions with **lactose intolerance** associated with **lactase deficiency**, Fig. 12.1.)

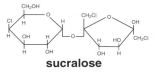

sucralose

Figure 12.3 Sucralose is a new sweetener made from sucrose by substituting three chlorine atoms for three hydroxyl groups. It is claimed to be poorly absorbed and not metabolised.

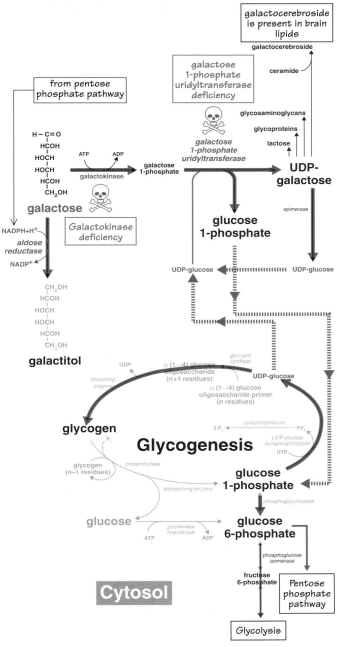

Figure 12.2 Galactose metabolism.

Oxidation/reduction reactions, coenzymes and prosthetic groups

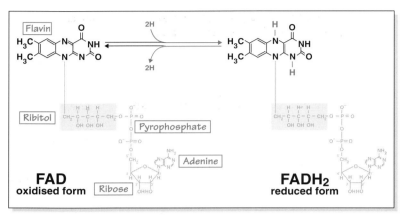

Figure 13.1 FAD (flavin adenine dinucleotide) is reduced to FADH₂.

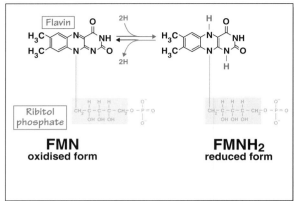

Figure 13.2 FMN (flavin mononucleotide) is reduced to FMNH₂.

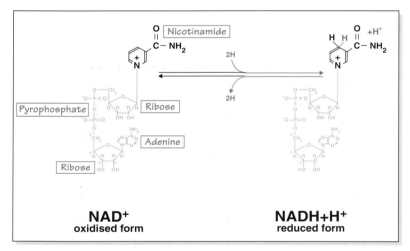

Figure 13.3 NAD⁺ (nicotinamide adenine dinucleotide) is reduced to NADH.

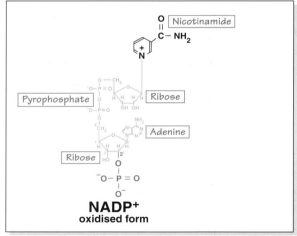

Figure 13.4 NADP⁺ (nicotinamide adenine dinucleotide phosphate) is similar to NAD⁺ except for the ribose 2′-phosphate moiety. Similarly, NADP⁺ is reduced to NADPH (not shown).

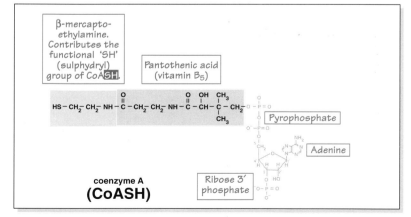

Figure 13.5 Coenzyme A. The SH (sulphydryl) group of β-mercaptoethylamine is the functional group which reacts, for example, with the carboxylate group of fatty acids.

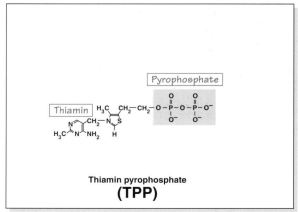

Figure 13.6 Thiamin pyrophosphate.

The hydrogen carriers: coenzymes: NAD⁺ and NADP⁺

NAD⁺ and **NADP⁺** (Figs 13.3 and 13.4) are coenzymes derived from niacin (Chapter 55) which function as co-substrates. Their job is to collaborate with enzyme X and collect the hydrogen from an oxidation reaction. In the process they are reduced to **NADH** and **NADPH**, respectively. Now, they say goodbye to enzyme X and diffuse away to collaborate with enzyme Y and donate hydrogen in a reducing reaction (in the process they are restored to their oxidised state: **NAD⁺** and **NADP⁺**).

NAD⁺ and NADP⁺, although very similar, have very different functions. **NADH is very important in energy metabolism** (e.g. Chapters 20 and 31) and **catabolic pathways**. **NADPH** is very important in **anabolic pathways** e.g. fatty acid synthesis (Chapter 23) and the "respiratory burst" (Chapter 18).

NB MAJOR CONCEPT: coenzymes such as NAD⁺, NADP⁺ and coenzyme A must be recycled (Fig. 13.7)! They are derived from vitamins, are present in tiny quantities and when reduced they must be *reoxidised in another enzyme reaction. Think of NAD⁺ and NADP⁺ as bees buzzing around the cell collecting hydrogen and then delivering it to a hydrogen user.*

Other coenzymes: coenzyme A and thiamine pyrophosphate

Coenzyme A and thiamine pyrophosphate are illustrated in Figs 13.5 and 13.6. For further details of other coenzymes see the chapters on vitamins (Chapter 55–58).

The prosthetic groups: FAD and FMN

FAD (Fig. 13.1) and **FMN** (Fig. 13.2) are enzyme co-factors derived from riboflavin (Chapter 55) and like NAD⁺ and NADP⁺ they collaborate as co-substrates in oxidation/reduction reactions and are reduced to **FADH₂** and **FMNH₂**. However, a major difference is that FAD and FMN are **not** coenzymes. They are **prosthetic groups**, meaning they are permanently attached to their enzymes by a covalent bond and therefore are a part of the enzyme structure.

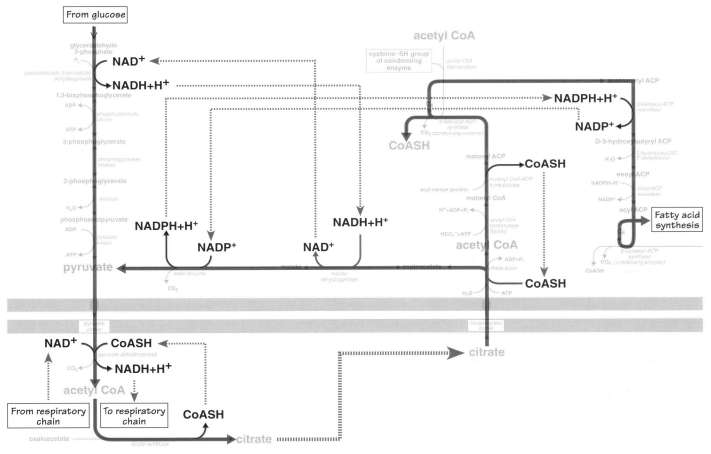

Figure 13.7 Coenzyme recycling. NAD⁺, NADP⁺ and coenzyme A (CoASH) are recycled in a partnership with another enzyme in the metabolic pathway. The pathway shown shows examples of coenzyme recycling when glucose is metabolised to fatty acids.

14
Anaerobic production of ATP by substrate-level phosphorylation, from phosphocreatine and by the adenylate kinase reaction

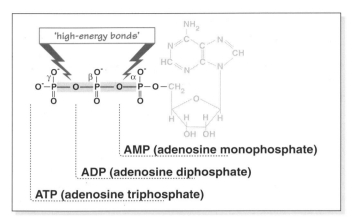

Figure 14.1 Structure of adenosine triphosphate (ATP).

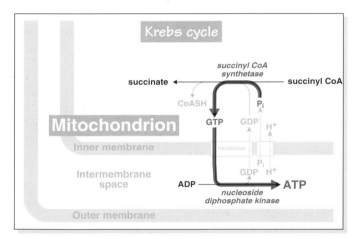

Figure 14.3 Substrate-level phosphorylation in Krebs cycle produces GTP which is converted to ATP.

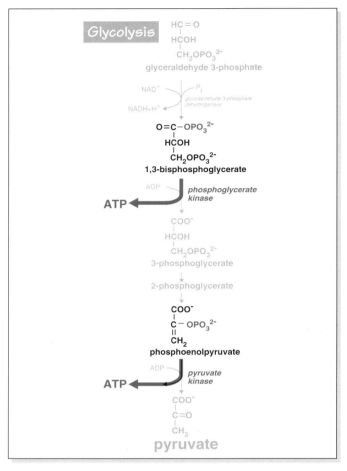

Figure 14.2 Substrate-level phosphorylation in glycolysis produces ATP.

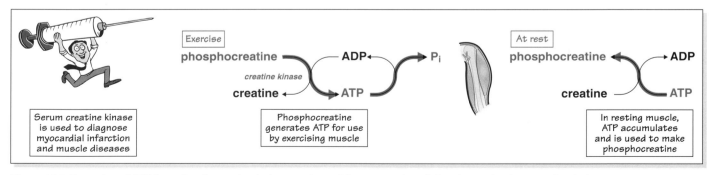

Figure 14.4 Formation of ATP from phosphocreatine during exercise and the regeneration of phosphocreatine from creatine during recovery.

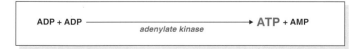

Figure 14.5 Formation of ATP from 2 molecules of ADP by the adenylate kinase reaction.

ATP (adenosine triphosphate): the molecule that provides energy for living cells

The ATP molecule is essential for life. It provides energy for muscle contraction, nerve conduction, many biochemical reactions, etc. At rest ATP turnover is 28 g (1 oz) of ATP per minute which is equivalent to 1.4 kg (3 lb) per hour. During strenuous exercise, ATP turnover increases to a massive 0.5 kg/min! Figure 14.1 shows that ATP consists of adenine, ribose and three phosphate groups which are identified as α-, β- and γ-. Hydrolysis of the "high-energy" **phosphoanhydride bonds** between the β- **and** γ-**phosphorus** atoms, or alternatively, between the α- **and** β-**phosphorus** atoms releases energy for the biochemical reactions of life.

Quantitatively, the most efficient method for producing ATP is by **aerobic** metabolism by oxidative phosphorylation (Chapters 20 and 31). However, ATP can also be produced albeit less efficiently under **anaerobic** conditions by **substrate-level phosphorylation**, from **phosphocreatine**, and by the **adenylate kinase reaction**. Although less efficient, the ability to produce ATP without oxygen can be of life-saving importance.

Production of ATP by substrate-level phosphorylation

Figure 14.2 shows that ATP is formed by the glycolytic reactions **phosphoglycerate kinase** and **pyruvate kinase**; and in Krebs cycle by **succinyl CoA synthetase** in co-operation with **nucleoside diphosphate kinase** (Fig. 14.3). *NB These reactions do not require oxygen.*

Production of ATP from phosphocreatine

Phosphocreatine is an important emergency reserve of "high-energy" phosphate which rapidly produces ATP for muscle contraction anaerobically. This can be of life-saving significance but, unfortunately, this supercharge mechanism for ATP production lasts only for a few seconds.

During periods of rest when ATP is abundant, **creatine** is phosphorylated by **creatine kinase** to form phosphocreatine. This reaction is especially important in muscles. When a sudden explosive burst of muscle activity occurs, phosphocreatine phosphorylates ADP to generate the ATP needed for muscle contraction (Fig. 14.4). For this reason, phosphocreatine is known as a "**phosphagen**".

Creatine is excreted as creatinine

Creatine is an amino acid but is not a component of proteins. It is made from arginine and is metabolised to **creatinine** prior to excretion in the urine (see Chapter 44). Blood levels of creatinine and the creatinine clearance test are used to evaluate glomerular filtration in renal disease.

*NB Do not be confused between **creatine**, **creatinine** and **carnitine**.*

Creatine as an ergogenic aid

Ergogenic aids are substances that enhance the speed, power or stamina of an athlete many of which are dangerous and illegal. Although controversial, a substantial body of opinion advocates **creatine** as the only ergogenic aid scientifically proven to enhance performance in both sprint and endurance events.

Production of ATP from ADP by adenylate kinase

When ATP has been hydrolysed to provide energy for muscle contraction, ADP accumulates. Remember that ADP still has a source of untapped energy in the α-phosphoanhydride bond (Fig. 14.1). With ingenious biochemical resourcefulness, this energy is salvaged when two molecules of ADP form ATP under anaerobic conditions using the **adenylate kinase** reaction (previously known as myokinase) (Fig. 14.5).

15 Aerobic production of ATP

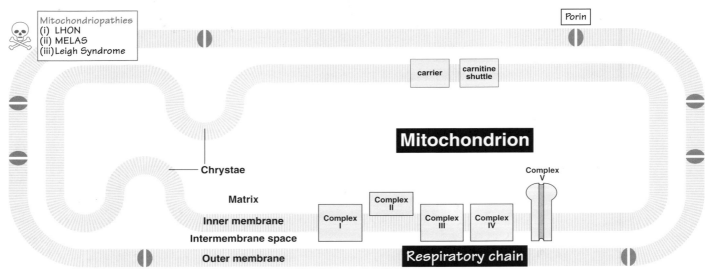

Figure 15.1 Diagram of a mitochondrion.

Production of ATP by oxidative phosphorylation in the respiratory chain

The mitochondrion

The mitochondrion (Fig. 15.1) is an organelle approximately the size of a bacterium. It is notable for having two membranes: an **outer membrane** that contains **porin** molecules rendering it permeable to molecules smaller than 10 kDa and an **inner membrane** that is **EXTREMELY IMPERMEABLE** and is folded into christae. Although small molecules such as H_2O and NH_3 can cross the inner membrane, carrier proteins and shuttle systems enable a few exclusive molecules to cross this barrier.

It is postulated that the inner membrane and its contents are derived from an ancient aerobic bacterium that invaded a primitive cell during the early stages of evolution and is an example of endosymbiosis. A relic from the past is that the mitochondrion has its own DNA (mtDNA) encoding 37 genes. Of these 24 are needed for mtDNA translation and the rest encode proteins of the respiratory chain. Notably only 13 of the more than 85 proteins composing the mitochondrial respiratory chain are encoded in mtDNA. The others are encoded by the nuclear DNA and imported from the cytoplasm.

The respiratory chain

The respiratory chain (Fig. 15.2 opposite) is a very efficient pathway for producing ATP from NADH and $FADH_2$, which in turn are formed by the oxidation of metabolic fuels, especially carbohydrates and fatty acids (Chapters 20 and 31). The respiratory chain consists of: complex I , complex II, complex III, complex IV and a mushroom-shaped multi-complex (complex V) comprising F_1 (fraction "one") and F_O (fraction "oh") that binds oligomycin. Some of these complexes contain cytochromes that transport electrons along the chain. Complex III contains cytochrome b, while complex IV contains cytochrome a/a3. Ubiquinone (coenzyme Q10) and cytochrome c also participate in electron transfer. The complexes are located in the mitochondrial inner membrane. Complexes I, III and IV not only transfer electrons but also pump protons into the intermembrane space. The inner membrane is very impermeable and in particular, it is impermeable to protons. The protons can return to the matrix only by passing through the F_1/F_0 complex, which generates ATP.

The flow of electrons is shown simplistically in Fig. 15.2. Chapter 16 illustrates how the flow of electrons (electric current) powers the proton pumps. Finally, the respiratory chain is shown in cartoon form in Figure 17.1.

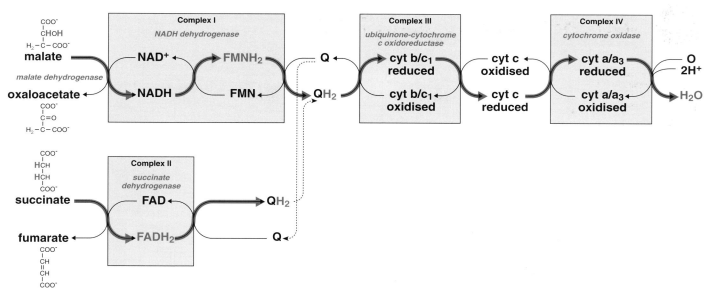

Figure 15.2 Electron transport in the respiratory chain. The diagram details the flow of electrons from the Krebs cycle intermediates malate and succinate via the electron transport chain (complexes I, II, III, IV) to oxygen.

Mitochondriopathies

There are several disorders of the respiratory chain. Many are transmitted by maternal inheritance as generally all mitochondria in the ovum are of maternal origin. The thousands of mtDNA molecules in one cell are distributed randomly to the daughter cells, therefore different tissues may harbour a mixture of both normal and mutant mtDNA (heteroplasmy). Accordingly the clinical phenotype is highly variable. Mutations in nuclear genes encoding proteins for the respiratory chain are transmitted autosomally and usually cause a more severe disease.

Leber hereditary optic neuropathy (LHON)

LHON is caused by a **mutation in the mitochondrial DNA** encoding one of the **complex I** subunits. It appears the optic nerve is expecially vulnerable to this respiratory chain dysfunction. This condition occurs in adults and results in loss of vision.

Mitochondrial encephalopathy, lactic acidosis and stroke-like episodes (MELAS)

MELAS is caused by a **mitochondrial DNA mutation** of the gene encoding leucine transfer RNA. This mutation affects translation of mitochondrial DNA so **all the respiratory chain complexes** are impaired with the exception of complex II which is totally encoded in the nucleus.

Leigh syndrome

Leigh syndrome is an early onset, degenerative, neurological disorder with characteristic neuropathological changes. Genetically, it is **heterogeneous** and is caused mainly by abnormal components of the respiratory chain encoded by **nuclear genes**; however, **mitochondrial gene abnormalities** also occur. The activity of **ATP synthetase (complex V) or complexes I, II, III and IV can be impaired**. There are also forms of Leigh syndrome that have **abnormal pyruvate dehydrogenase complex (PDH)** activity (Chapter 30).

PDH deficiency results in raised blood concentrations of pyruvate, lactate and alanine. Some patients respond to supplementation with lipoic acid or thiamine (coenzymes for PDH). Treatment with a low carbohydrate, ketogenic diet has been advocated but with limited success. *(The ketone bodies readily cross the blood brain barrier and their catabolism produces acetyl CoA independently of PDH.)*

The biosynthesis of ATP by oxidative phosphorylation II

17

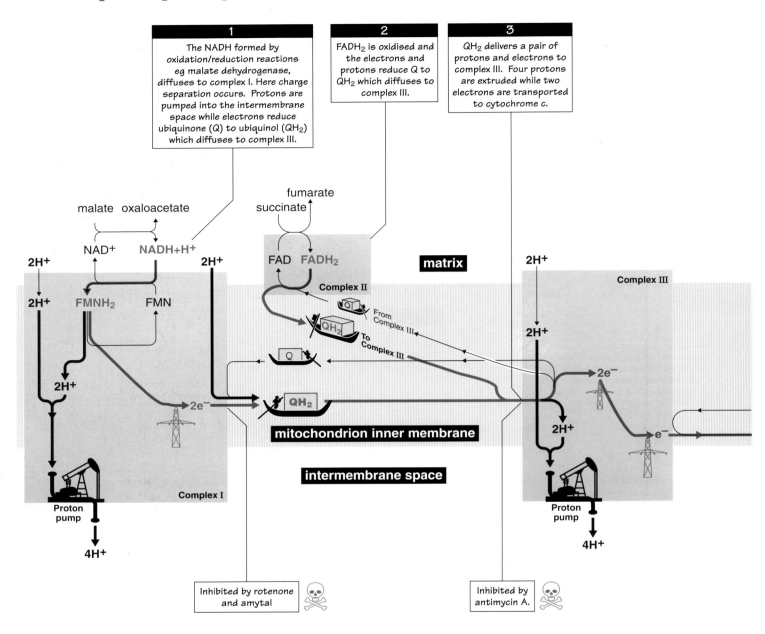

1
The NADH formed by oxidation/reduction reactions eg malate dehydrogenase, diffuses to complex I. Here charge separation occurs. Protons are pumped into the intermembrane space while electrons reduce ubiquinone (Q) to ubiquinol (QH_2) which diffuses to complex III.

2
$FADH_2$ is oxidised and the electrons and protons reduce Q to QH_2 which diffuses to complex III.

3
QH_2 delivers a pair of protons and electrons to complex III. Four protons are extruded while two electrons are transported to cytochrome c.

malate   oxaloacetate

NAD^+ $NADH+H^+$

$2H^+$

$2H^+$

$FMNH_2$ FMN

$2H^+$

$2e^-$

Proton pump

Complex I

$4H^+$

Inhibited by rotenone and amytal

$2H^+$

fumarate
succinate

FAD $FADH_2$

matrix

Complex II

From Complex III

QH_2

To Complex III

QH_2

mitochondrion inner membrane

intermembrane space

$2H^+$

$2H^+$

Complex III

$2H^+$

$2e^-$

$2H^+$

e^-

Proton pump

$4H^+$

Inhibited by antimycin A.

The flow of electrons and protons from **NADH⁺** and **FADH₂** via **complexes I** and **II** respectively, to **complex III** of the respiratory chain are shown in Fig. 17.1. Electrons are then transported to **complex IV** where they combine with oxygen. Meanwhile, protons are pumped into the intermembrane space and are returned to the matrix via the proton channel in the **Fₒ** subunit of the ATP synthetase (complex V). The flow of protons ("protonicity") drives a molecular motor in the **ATP synthetase** complex (F₁ particle) which aligns molecules of **ADP** and **Pi** so they combine to form **ATP**.

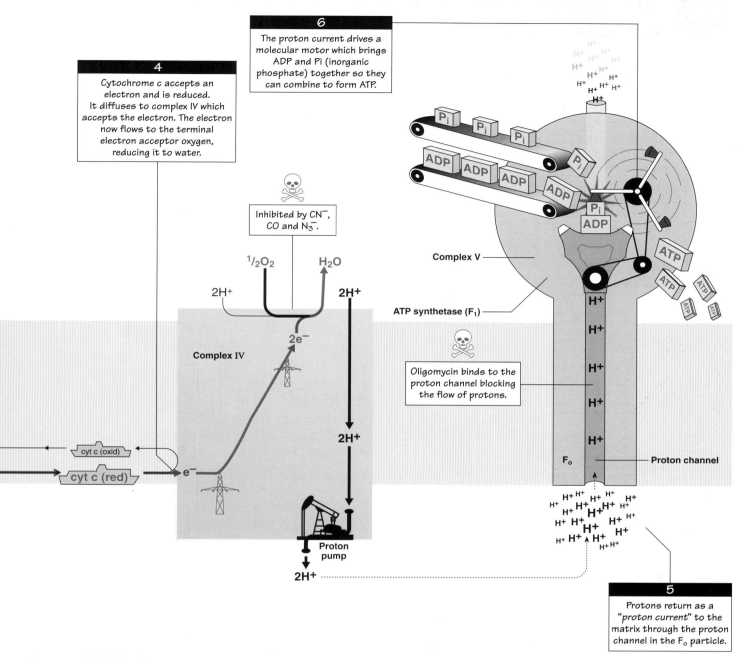

4

Cytochrome c accepts an electron and is reduced. It diffuses to complex IV which accepts the electron. The electron now flows to the terminal electron acceptor oxygen, reducing it to water.

6

The proton current drives a molecular motor which brings ADP and Pi (inorganic phosphate) together so they can combine to form ATP.

Inhibited by CN^-, CO and N_3^-.

$^1/_2O_2$ H_2O

$2H^+$ $2H^+$

$2e^-$

Complex IV

$2H^+$

cyt c (oxid)

cyt c (red)

e^-

Proton pump

$2H^+$

P_i P_i P_i

ADP ADP ADP

P_i

ADP

P_i
ADP

ATP

Complex V

ATP synthetase (F_1)

H^+

H^+

H^+

H^+

H^+

Oligomycin binds to the proton channel blocking the flow of protons.

F_o **Proton channel**

H^+ ...

5

Protons return as a "proton current" to the matrix through the proton channel in the F_o particle.

Figure 17.1 Oxidative phosphorylation. A cartoon representation of electron and proton transport via the respiratory chain which produces ATP by oxidative phosphorylation. A concise version of this diagram which is more appropriate for examination purposes is in Chapter 15.

18 What happens when protons or electrons leak from the respiratory chain?

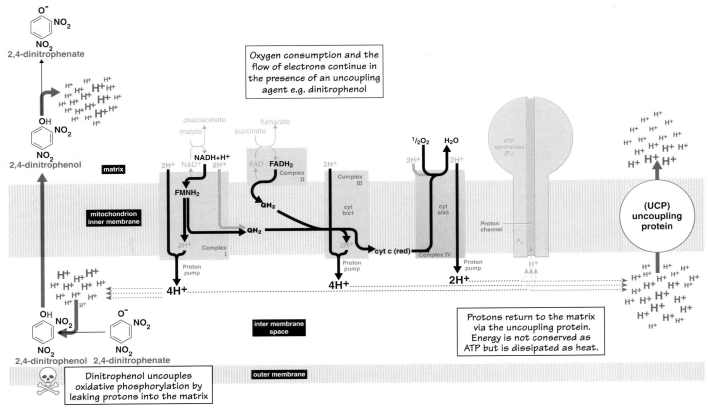

Figure 18.1 Dinitrophenol and uncoupling protein uncouple oxidative phosphorylation from electron transport.

Leakage of protons or electrons from the respiratory chain

We have seen in the previous pages how the formation of ATP from ADP by oxidative phosphorylation depends on both a flow of protons (a proton current) and a flow of electrons (an electron current). Inevitably there will be consequences if either proton or electron leakage occurs. **Proton leakage is associated with thermogenesis. Electron leakage is associated with the formation of reactive oxygen species (ROS)** which can be extremely toxic.

Proton leakage and thermogenesis
Dinitrophenol (DNP)

During World War 1, workers in the munitions factories developed fevers and lost weight. This was later attributed to the explosive they were handling called dinitrophenol (**DNP**). The ability of DNP to "speed up the metabolic rate" was exploited as a slimming pill until it was banned in the 1930s because of its adverse side effects. DNP causes

protons to leak from the intermembrane space to the matrix thus bypassing the **ATP synthetase** system (Fig. 18.1).

DNP is an "uncoupling agent" and **uncouples electron transport from oxidative phosphorylation**. It does this when the **dinitrophenolate anion** accepts a proton to form **dinitrophenol**, which is lipid soluble, and diffuses across the mitochondrial inner membrane. When it reaches the matrix, it dissociates releasing its proton. The energy which otherwise would have been used for ATP synthesis is dissipated as heat (hence the fevers experienced by the munitions workers).

Uncoupling protein

Uncoupling protein 1 (UCP1) (originally called **thermogenin**) is found only in mammalian brown adipose tissue and is responsible for cold-induced, non-shivering thermogenesis. It performs this function by enabling protons to leak from the intermembrane space into the matrix with the energy being dissipated as heat (Fig. 18.1).

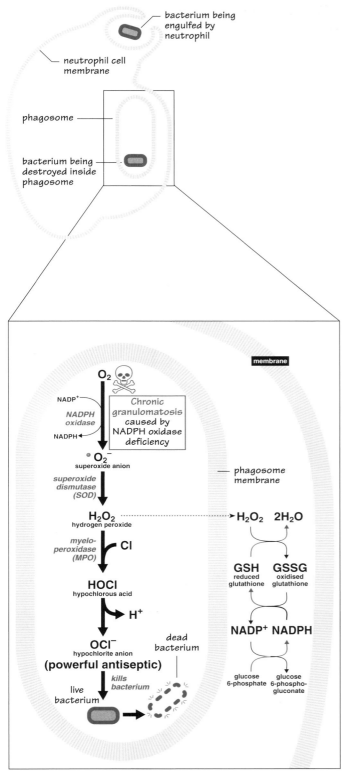

bacterium being
engulfed by
neutrophil

neutrophil cell
membrane

phagosome

bacterium being
destroyed inside
phagosome

membrane

O₂

NADP⁺

**NADPH
oxidase**

NADPH

Chronic
granulomatosis
caused by
NADPH oxidase
deficiency

$^•O_2^-$
superoxide anion

*superoxide
dismutase
(SOD)*

phagosome
membrane

H_2O_2
hydrogen peroxide

H_2O_2 $2H_2O$

*myelo-
peroxidase
(MPO)*   Cl

GSH   GSSG
reduced   oxidised
glutathione   glutathione

HOCl
hypochlorous acid

H⁺

NADP⁺ NADPH

OCl⁻
hypochlorite anion

dead
bacterium

(powerful antiseptic)

glucose
6-phosphate

glucose
6-phospho-
gluconate

live
bacterium

*kills
bacterium*

Figure 18.2 The respiratory burst in phagocytes kills bacteria.

Leakage of electrons from the respiratory chain produces reactive oxygen species (ROS)

ROS are extremely toxic and a more detailed description of their production and devastating effects is provided in Chapter 19. (*Readers might prefer to study Chapter 19 before returning to this text.*)

The respiratory chain is the major source of ROS

In theory, molecular oxygen should be **completely reduced** in complex IV by four electrons to form water without the formation of intermediates. **In practice**, occasionally **partial reduction** occurs with oxygen being converted to **superoxide anion radicals** (Chapter 19). Also, the ubiquinone reactions in complex I and complex II have an unfortunate tendency to leak electrons directly to oxygen. Overall up to 2% of cellular oxygen forms superoxide free radicals and the body has developed defence mechanisms such as **superoxide dismutase**, **glutathione reductase** and **catalase** to dispose of them.

ROS as "good guys": the "respiratory burst" makes bleach!

Although ROS are extremely toxic, this can be used to the body's advantage as exemplified by the "respiratory burst". The respiratory burst is a sudden surge of aerobic metabolism producing **hypochlorous acid** which is used to kill pathogens (Fig. 18.2).

Phagocytic cells such as macrophages and neutrophils defend the body against pathogens with microbiocidal peptides and lytic enzymes. They also produce microbiocidal oxidants whose formation is accompanied by a transient episode of oxidative metabolism known as the "**respiratory burst**" (see Fig. 18.2 and Fig. 19.1 for more details). The neutrophil engulfs the pathogen in a membrane-enclosed phagosome and **NADPH oxidase** is activated on the phagosomal membrane producing **superoxide anions**. These are converted to oxygen and hydrogen peroxide by **superoxide dismutase (SOD)**. In neutrophils (but not macrophages), **myeloperoxidase** catalyses the oxidation of chloride ions by hydrogen peroxide forming **hypochlorous acid** (yes, the swimming pool sanitiser and domestic bleach!) and this dissociates forming **hypochlorite ions**, which kill the pathogens.

Chronic granulomatous disease (CGD) is a rare, X-linked deficiency of NADPH oxidase activity which drastically impairs the ability of macrophages and neutrophils to destroy pathogens. Patients are especially vulnerable to infection by *Mycobacteria*, *Escherichia coli* and *Staphylococci* since these organisms produce catalase to defend themselves against hydrogen peroxide attack by the phagocytes.

19 Free radicals, reactive oxygen species and oxidative damage

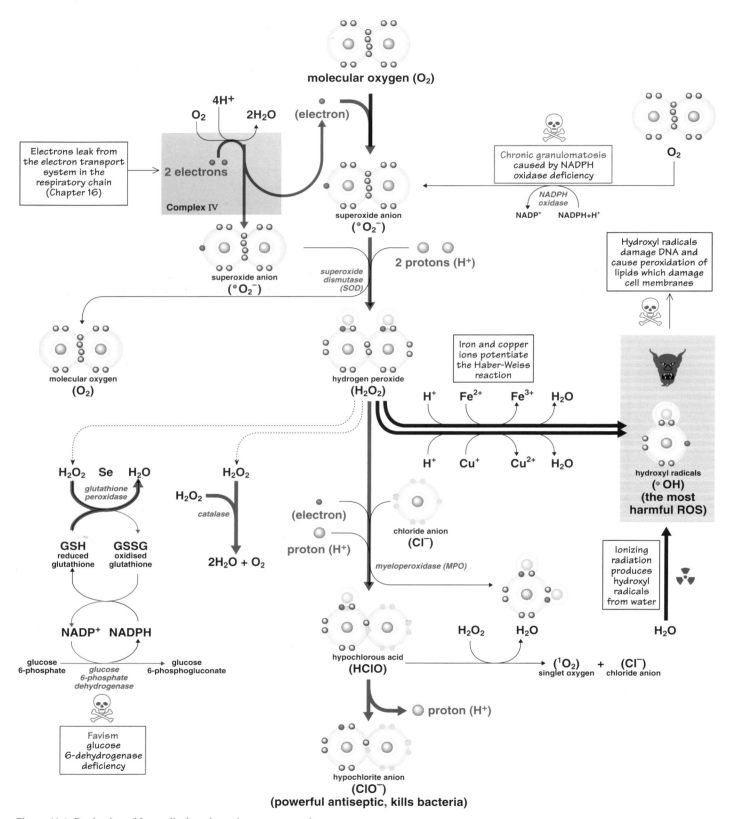

Figure 19.1 Production of free radicals and reactive oxygen species.

Reactive oxygen species (ROS) and free radicals

Reactive oxygen species (ROS) is a term which describes: (i) **free radicals**, e.g. the hydroxyl radical $\cdot OH$ (NB it differs from the hydroxyl ion OH^-), (ii) **ions**, e.g. the hypochlorite ion ClO^- the conjugate base formed from the dissociation of hypochlorous acid and the active component of domestic bleach; (iii) **a combined free radical and ion**, e.g. the superoxide anion $\cdot O_2^-$ or (iv) **molecules**, e.g. hydrogen peroxide H_2O_2.

A free radical is any species capable of independent existence with at least one unpaired electron (shown as $\cdot$) in its outer orbit. Particularly prone are unsaturated fats leading to the process of lipid peroxidation. Free radicals are very unstable, short-lived molecules which react rapidly with adjacent molecules causing cellular damage. They do this by stealing an electron from a neighbouring molecule to partner its own unpaired electron. That would be fine except that the neighbouring molecule now has a lone electron and has become a free radical! A breakdown of molecular law and order results in a chain reaction of neighbour stealing an electron from its neighbour, and the result can be damage to the cell.

Production of free radicals
Respiratory chain
The respiratory chain is the major source of oxygen free radicals. **In theory**, molecular oxygen should be completely reduced in complex IV by four electrons from water without the formation of intermediates. **In practice**, sometimes partial reduction occurs with oxygen being converted to superoxide anion radicals. Also, the ubiquinone reactions in complex I and complex II have an unfortunate tendency to leak electrons directly to oxygen. Overall up to 2% of cellular oxygen forms superoxide free radicals and the body has developed defence mechanisms to counter their damaging effects.

Ionising radiation
The interaction of ionising radiation with H_2O and O_2 generates free radicals. However, although they can be harmful to normal cells, during radiotherapy when they are focused on cancer cells in a high-dose target zone, lethal free-radical-mediated damage to the cancer cell DNA occurs.

Pollutants
Tobacco smoke contains epoxides and peroxides that may react with and damage the alveoli. The tar contains free radicals derived from quinones and semiquinones. Inhalation of inorganic particles such as asbestos causes free-radical-mediated lung damage.

Myocardial ischaemia and reperfusion-induced injury
Reperfusion to restore the flow of oxygenated blood to ischaemic tissue is essential for its survival but it produces oxygen free radicals, which are thought to be responsible for reperfusion-induced injury.

Metal ions
The transition metals, especially copper and iron ions, catalyse the formation of the dreaded hydroxyl radicals ($\cdot OH$) from hydrogen peroxide (Haber-Weiss reaction). Because iron mediates oxidative damage, the substantial intracellular pool of free iron must be regulated by iron chelators, e.g. intracellular storage proteins such as ferritin.

Free radicals: friend or foe?
Free radicals as friends
Free radicals are not always the bad guys! **Nitric oxide** ($NO\cdot$) is produced by the endothelial cells to control blood pressure, **hydrogen peroxide** is needed to make thyroxine, and phagocytes produce **ROS** which kill pathogens using the **respiratory burst** (Chapter 18).

Free radicals as foes
Free radicals usually are bad guys. They cause peroxidation damage to lipids, damage DNA causing cancer and inflict oxidative damage on the body's tissues, contributing to premature ageing and many degenerative diseases especially cardiovascular disease. The most harmful are hydroxyl radicals ($\cdot OH$).

Defence mechanisms against free radicals and reactive oxygen species
Enzymic defences
As shown in Fig. 19.1, **superoxide dismutase (SOD)**, dismutes superoxide anions to hydrogen peroxide, which is safely converted to water and molecular oxygen by **catalase**. Furthermore, hydrogen peroxide is disposed of by cytosolic **glutathione peroxidase**, a **selenium**-dependant enzyme that provides a major route for elimination.

Free radical scavengers
Free radical scavengers are molecules that react with free radicals and render them harmless. There is considerable interest in foods rich in vitamins A, C and E (Chapters 53, 54 and 58) and those with an abundance of phytochemicals such as the phenols, polyphenols and flavonoids which have high oxygen radical absorbance capacity (ORAC) values. These are potent free radical scavengers which are thought to reduce the risk of several chronic degenerative disorders.

Oxygen radical absorbance capacity (ORAC) values
Recently there has been popular interest in the beneficial effects of foods with high ORAC values. ORAC values are an assessment of the total antioxidant content of foods (including, for example, phenols, and vitamins C and E) assessed as mMol TE/kg, where TE is "Trolox equivalent". Trolox® is a water-soluble, analogue of vitamin E with potent antioxidant properties used as a reference compound for the *in vitro* food tests.

Aerobic oxidation of glucose to provide energy as ATP

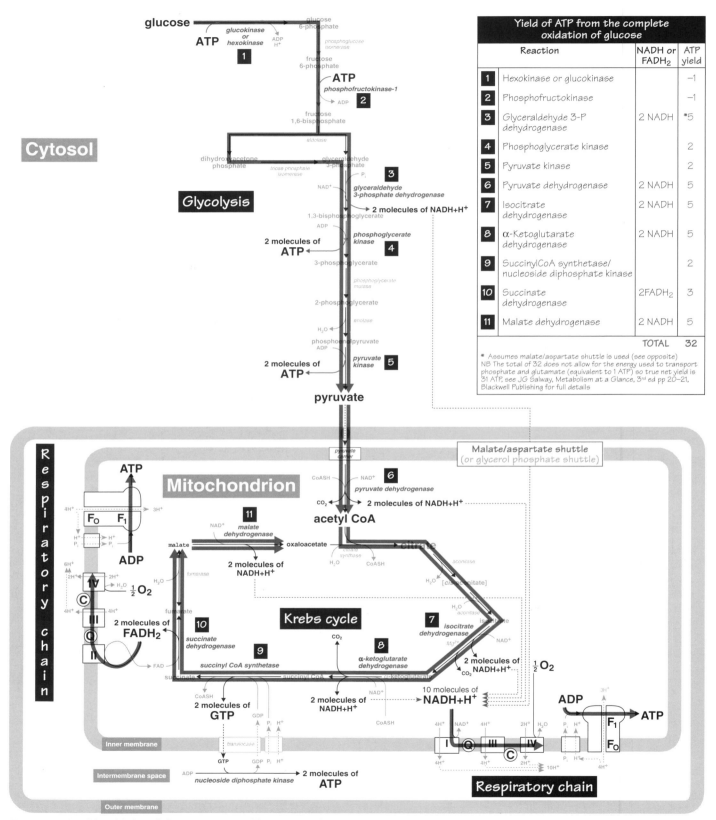

	Reaction	NADH or FADH$_2$	ATP yield
1	Hexokinase or glucokinase		−1
2	Phosphofructokinase		−1
3	Glyceraldehyde 3-P dehydrogenase	2 NADH	*5
4	Phosphoglycerate kinase		2
5	Pyruvate kinase		2
6	Pyruvate dehydrogenase	2 NADH	5
7	Isocitrate dehydrogenase	2 NADH	5
8	α-Ketoglutarate dehydrogenase	2 NADH	5
9	SuccinylCoA synthetase/ nucleoside diphosphate kinase		2
10	Succinate dehydrogenase	2FADH$_2$	3
11	Malate dehydrogenase	2 NADH	5
		TOTAL	32

* Assumes malate/aspartate shuttle is used (see opposite)
NB The total of 32 does not allow for the energy used to transport phosphate and glutamate (equivalent to 1 ATP) so true net yield is 31 ATP, see JG Salway, Metabolism at a Glance, 3rd ed pp 20–21, Blackwell Publishing for full details

Figure 20.1 Aerobic oxidation of glucose to generate 32 molecules of ATP.

The malate/aspartate shuttle and the glycerol 3-phosphate shuttle

How does NADH cross the mitochondrial inner membrane? The NADH produced by glyceraldehyde 3-phosphate dehydrogenase must enter the mitochondrion before it can be used to produce ATP. Problem: the inner membrane of the mitochondrial membrane is impermeable to NADH. The problem is overcome by processes that transfer the electrons (and protons) from NADH to malate or glycerol 3-phosphate, namely the malate/aspartate shuttle or the glycerol 3-phosphate shuttle.

Malate/aspartate shuttle. Cytosolic malate dehydrogenase transfers the electrons and protons from **NADH** to **oxaloacetate** forming **malate**. Malate enters the mitochondrion via the **dicarboxylate carrier** in exchange for **α-ketoglutarate**. **Mitochondrial malate dehydroge-**

nase transfers the electrons and protons to NAD⁺ forming **oxaloacetate** and **NADH** which generates **2.5 molecules of ATP** in the respiratory chain. To complete the cycle, oxaloacetate is transaminated to aspartate which enters the cytosol and is converted back to oxaloacetate.

Glycerol 3-phosphate shuttle. **Cytosolic glyceraldehyde 3-phosphate dehydrogenase** transfers the electrons and protons from **NADH** to **dihydroxyacetone phosphate** forming **glycerol 3-phosphate**. **Mitochondrial glycerol 3-phosphate dehydrogenase** in the inner membrane transfers electrons and protons to its prosthetic group **FAD** forming **FADH₂**, which passes to the respiratory chain and generates **1.5 molecules of ATP**. This reaction also generates dihydroxyacetone phosphate which completes the cycle.

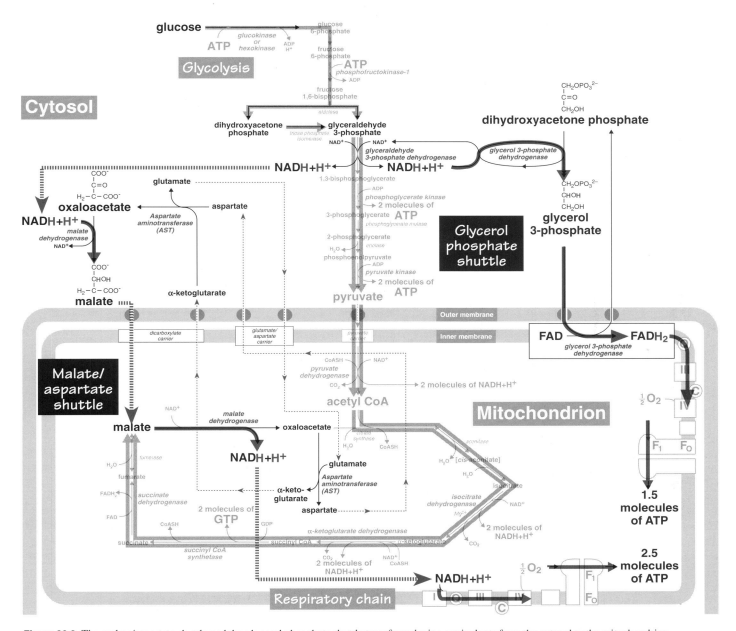

Figure 20.2 The malate/aspartate shuttle and the glycerol phosphate shuttle transfer reducing equivalents from the cytosol to the mitochondrion.

Anaerobic oxidation of glucose by glycolysis to form ATP and lactate

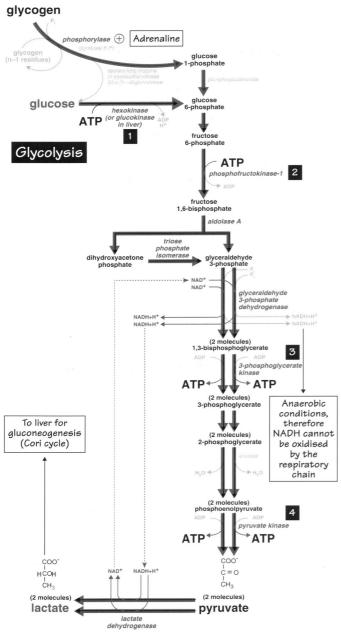

Figure 21.1 Anaerobic metabolism of glucose and glycogen to generate ATP.

Anaerobic glycolysis

Glucose can be metabolised to generate a **net total of 2 molecules of ATP** in the absence of oxygen, i.e. **anaerobically** (Fig. 21.1). As shown in Table 21.1, this initially needs the **investment** of ATP for each of the **hexokinase** and **phosphofructokinase** reactions. **Fructose 6-phosphate** is eventually split into **2** molecules of **glyceraldehyde 3-phosphate** which when oxidised by **glyceraldehyde 3-phosphate dehydrogenase** yields **2 NADH**. **Two** molecules of **ATP** are produced by phosphoglycerate kinase and another **2 molecules** of **ATP** are made in the **pyruvate kinase** reaction. *NB Under **aerobic conditions**, NADH is oxidised by the respiratory chain to recycle NAD⁺ for the glyceraldehyde 3-phosphate dehydrogenase reaction. (Remember that NAD⁺ and NADH are present in small amounts and must always be recycled.)* However, under **anaerobic** conditions **lactate dehydrogenase** causes NADH to reduce pyruvate and NAD⁺ is recycled for **glyceraldehyde 3-phosphate dehydrogenase**. The lactate goes to the liver and forms glucose by gluconeogenesis in the **Cori cycle** (Fig. 21.2).

Note that when glycogen is the source of glucose 6-phosphate, the net yield is **3 molecules of ATP** (Table 21.2).

Table 21.1 Anaerobic glycolysis from glucose yields 2 molecules of ATP.

Yield of ATP from the anaerobic oxidation of glucose to lactate		
Reaction	NADH or FADH₂	ATP yield
1 Hexokinase (or glucokinase in liver)		−1
2 Phosphofructokinase-1		−1
3 3-Phosphoglycerate kinase		2
4 Pyruvate kinase		2
	TOTAL	2

Table 21.2 Anaerobic glycolysis from glycogen yields 3 molecules of ATP.

Yield of ATP from the anaerobic oxidation of a glucose residue derived from glycogen to lactate		
Reaction	NADH or FADH₂	ATP yield
2 Phosphofructokinase-1		−1
3 3-Phosphoglycerate kinase		2
4 Pyruvate kinase		2
	TOTAL	3

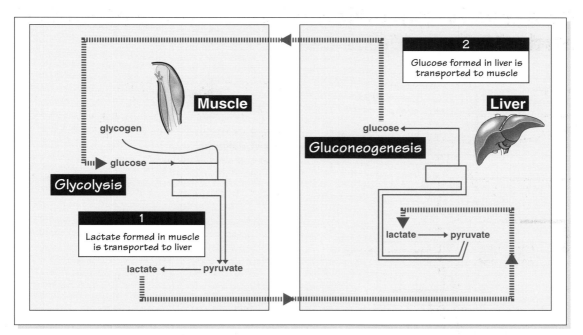

Figure 21.2 The Cori cycle. Glucose consumed by the liver is metabolised to lactate. This lactate is converted to glucose in the liver and recycled to muscle.

The fate of the lactate: Cori cycle

Lactate is being produced continuously from glucose by anaerobic glycolysis in red blood cells, the retina and the kidney medulla. This lactate is recycled to glucose by a process known as the Cori cycle. The lactate is returned to the liver and is metabolised to glucose by **gluconeogenesis** in a process that consumes the equivalent of 6 molecules of ATP (Chapter 32). If the Cori cycle is interrupted by liver disease, lactate accumulates resulting in hyperlactataemia. Asymptomatic hyperlactataemia is a benign condition that is fairly common and rarely progresses to life-threatening lactic acidosis which overwhelms the body's buffer systems.

22 Anaerobic glycolysis in red blood cells, 2,3-BPG and the Bohr effect

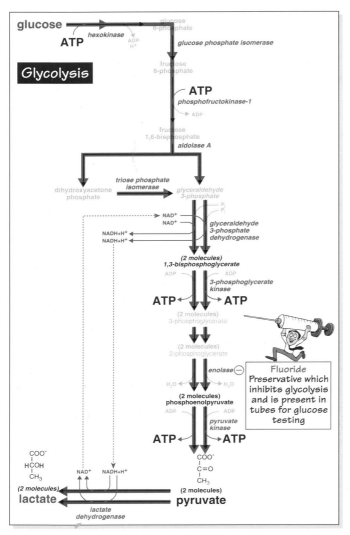

Figure 22.1 Anaerobic glycolysis in the red blood cell.

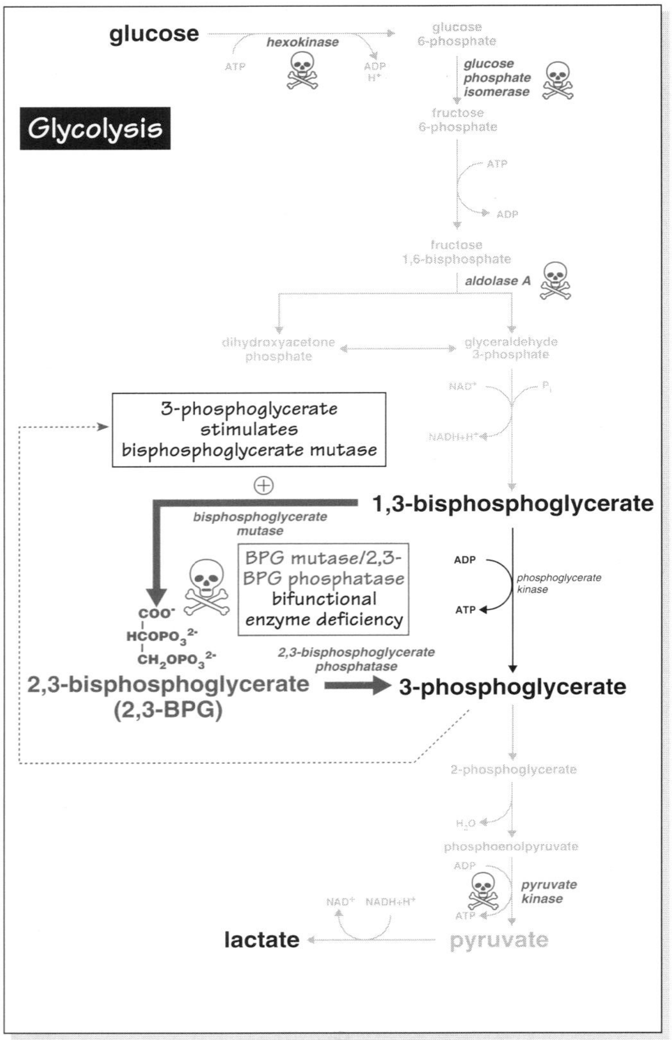

Figure 22.2 Production of 2,3-bisphosphoglycerate in the red blood cell.

The red blood cells contain an abundance of oxygen which they transport around the body, but ironically they cannot use this oxygen themselves and are entirely dependent on glucose for fuel by **anaerobic** glycolysis to produce ATP (Fig. 22.1). This is because they lack mitochondria and consequently the enzymes for Krebs cycle. Similarly, red blood cells also lack the enzymes for fatty acid oxidation and ketone body utilisation.

The function of red blood cells is to transport oxygen, which they do by binding oxygen tightly to form **oxyhaemoglobin**. The problem is that when the red cells arrive at the peripheral tissue, they must be persuaded to unload their cargo of oxygen. They achieve this by the phenomenon known as the **Bohr effect**, which involves two contributing factors: **protons** and **2,3-bisphosphoglycerate** as shown in Fig. 22.2.

1. Protons displace oxygen from oxyhaemoglobin. The production of ATP in exercising muscle involves Krebs cycle which produces

carbon dioxide. Carbon dioxide enters the red cell where **carbonic anhydrase** catalyses its reaction with water to form **carbonic acid**. Carbonic acid decomposes spontaneously to **bicarbonate** and results in a localised **increase in the concentration of protons [H⁺]** (i.e. a decrease in pH). These protons release oxygen from haemoglobin. The oxygen then diffuses from the red cell into the peripheral tissues where it binds to myoglobin, which transports the oxygen to the respiratory chain where it is used to produce ATP by oxidative phosphorylation. (The carbonic anhydrase reaction is described in a different context in Chapters 3–5.)

2. Unloading oxygen in the periphery: 2,3-bisphosphoglycerate (2,3-BPG) stabilises deoxyhaemoglobin. The other factor is 2,3-BPG (Fig. 22.2), which is better known in clinical circles as **2,3-diphosphoglycerate (2,3-DPG)**. The 2,3-BPG is formed under anoxic conditions in red blood cells by the 2,3-BPG shunt (**Rapoport–Luebering**

shunt) (Fig. 22.2). In the peripheral tissues, a molecule of 2,3-BPG binds to **deoxyhaemoglobin** which stabilises the structure and prevents it from grabbing hold of oxygen from adjacent molecules of **oxyhaemoglobin**.

3. Loading oxygen in the lungs. The red blood cells transport **deoxyhaemoglobin** and its cargo of CO_2 to the lungs. In the lungs there is a high partial pressure of oxygen that displaces the CO_2 which is exhaled from the lungs. Now oxygen binds to form **oxyhaemoglobin** 2,3-BPG is displaced and the red cell proceeds to the periphery with its new load of oxygen.

2,3-BPG in health and disease
Fetal haemoglobin has a low affinity for 2,3-BPG
Haemoglobin is a tetramer of two α-chains and two β-chains. However, fetal haemoglobin consists of two α-chains and two γ-chains. Fetal haemoglobin has a lower affinity for 2,3-BPG than adult haemoglobin. This means that fetal haemoglobin has an affinity for oxygen that is greater than the maternal haemoglobin and this facilitates oxygen transfer from the mother to the fetus.

2,3-BPG and adaptation to high altitude
Anyone who lives at low altitude who has flown to a high-altitude location knows that even moderate exertion can cause breathlessness. Within a few days adaptation occurs as the concentration of 2,3-BPG in the red cells increases, enabling the tissues to obtain oxygen despite its relatively diminished availability in the thin mountain air.

Increased 2,3-BPG is the body's response to a lack of oxygen
The concentration of 2,3-BPG is increased in smokers, which compensates for a diminished oxygen supply because of their chronic exposure to carbon monoxide. Also, a compensatory increase in 2,3-BPG is commonly seen in patients with chronic anaemia, obstructive lung disease, congenital heart disease and cystic fibrosis.

Red cell enzymopathies of the glycolytic pathway
Inherited diseases due to deficiency of red cell glycolytic enzymes are rare causes of hereditary, non-spherocytic haemolytic anaemia. This can be serious for two reasons as the red cell is entirely dependent on glycolysis for production of: (i) ATP and (ii) 2,3-BPG.

The effect on 2,3-BPG metabolism varies (Fig. 22.2). If the disorder is **proximal** to the **2,3-BPG shunt** (e.g. deficiencies of **hexokinase, phosphoglucose isomerase** and **aldolase A)**, the flow of metabolites through glycolysis will be decreased and consequently the concentration of 2,3-BPG will **fall**. If the deficiency is **distal** to the **2,3-BPG shunt** (e.g. **pyruvate kinase** deficiency) the concentration of 2,3-BPG will **rise**.

Finally, patients have been reported with deficiency of the bifunctional shunt enzyme, **BPG mutase/2,3-BPG phosphatase** and these patients have low concentrations of 2,3-BPG.

Aldolase nomenclature
This can be confusing! Aldolase (full name: fructose 1,6-bisphosphate aldolase) is officially known as D-glyceraldehyde 3-phosphate lyase, EC 4.1.2.13). It has three functions:
(1) It catalyses the condensation of dihydroxyacetone phosphate with glyceraldehyde 3-phosphate to form fructose 1,6-bisphosphate.
(2) It catalyses the splitting of fructose 1,6-bisphosphate to dihydroxyacetone phosphate and glyceraldehyde 3-phosphate.
(3) It catalyses the cleavage of structurally similar sugar phosphates e.g. fructose 1-phosphate to dihydroxyacetone phosphate and glyceraldehyde (Chapter 24). (*NB This function was previously described as ketose phosphate 1-aldolase, EC 4.1.2.7*).
In animals three forms of aldolase have been described:
Aldolase A. In blood a defective form of aldolase A is present in hereditary haemolytic anaemia (Fig. 22.2). Aldolase A also occurs in muscle.
Aldolase B. Deficiency of aldolase B causes hereditary fructose intolerance (Chapter 24). Aldolase B occurs in liver, kidney and small intestine.
Aldolase C. Occurs in brain.

23 The fate of glucose in liver: glycogenesis and lipogenesis

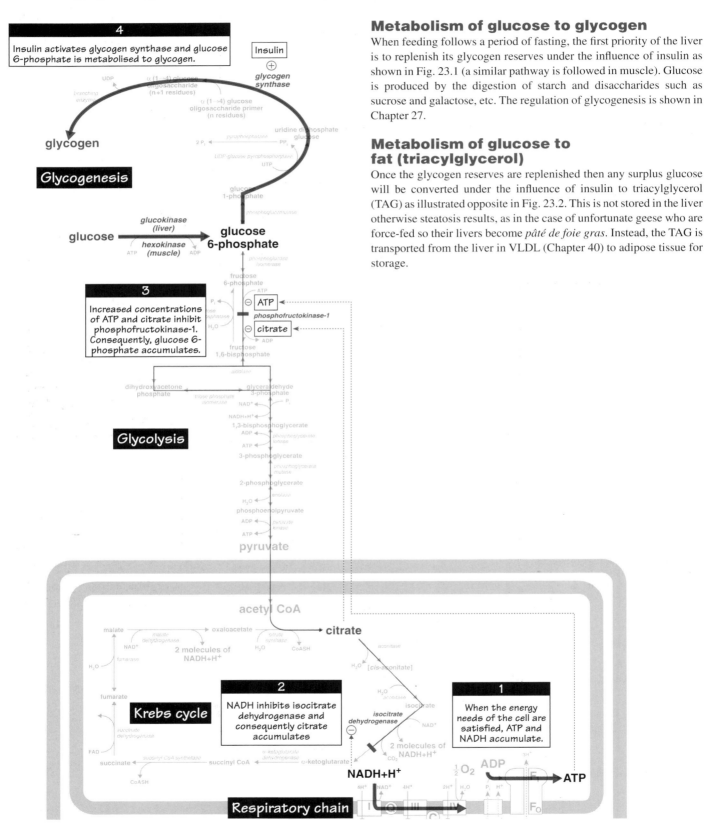

Metabolism of glucose to glycogen

When feeding follows a period of fasting, the first priority of the liver is to replenish its glycogen reserves under the influence of insulin as shown in Fig. 23.1 (a similar pathway is followed in muscle). Glucose is produced by the digestion of starch and disaccharides such as sucrose and galactose, etc. The regulation of glycogenesis is shown in Chapter 27.

Metabolism of glucose to fat (triacylglycerol)

Once the glycogen reserves are replenished then any surplus glucose will be converted under the influence of insulin to triacylglycerol (TAG) as illustrated opposite in Fig. 23.2. This is not stored in the liver otherwise steatosis results, as in the case of unfortunate geese who are force-fed so their livers become *pâté de foie gras*. Instead, the TAG is transported from the liver in VLDL (Chapter 40) to adipose tissue for storage.

Figure 23.1 Metabolism of glucose to glycogen in liver.

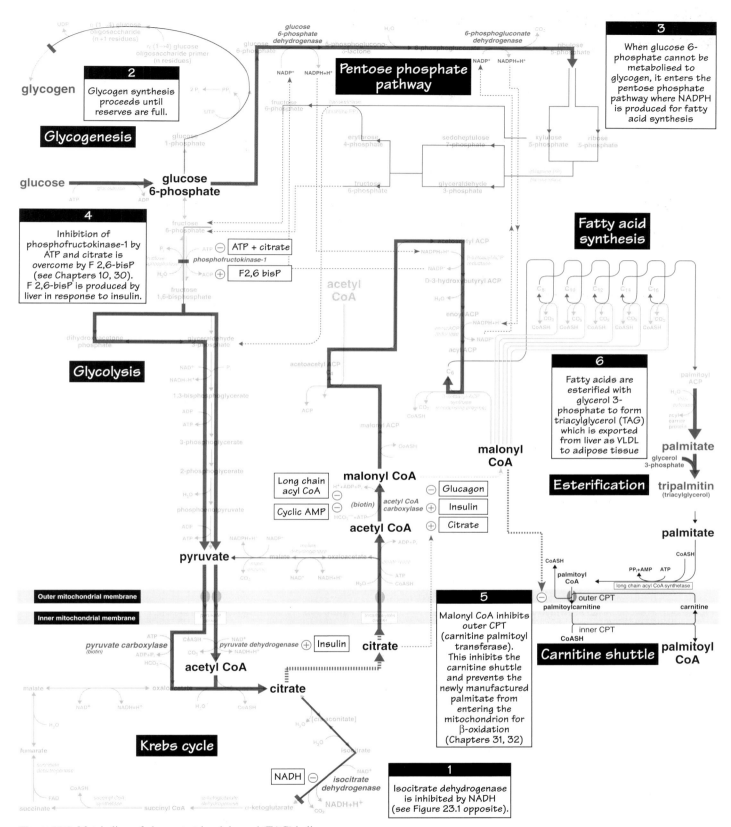

Figure 23.2 Metabolism of glucose to triacylglycerol (TAG) in liver.

Glucose homeostasis

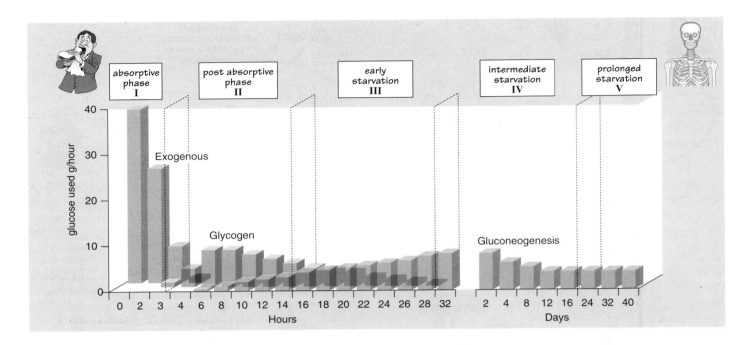

Figure 25.1 Rate of glucose utilisation during the five phases of glucose homeostasis. (Adapted from: Ruderman NB (1975) Muscle amino acid metabolism and gluconeogenesis. *Annu Rev Med* **26**, 245–58. © 1975 Annual Reviews www.annualreviews.org. with permission.)

The importance of glucose homeostasis

The fasting blood glucose concentration is normally maintained between 3.5 and 5.5 mMol/l. After a meal, the blood glucose concentration normally rises briefly above 5.5 mMol/l up to about 9 mMol/l but within 2 hours it will return to the fasting level. Conversely, it is a remarkable fact that the body normally is capable of maintaining the blood glucose concentration above 3.5 mMol/l despite the challenges of prolonged starvation or strenuous exercise. For example, glucose homeostasis is maintained despite the sudden massive demand for glucose made by an athletic sprinter or by a Marathon runner. If this did not happen, the blood glucose concentration would fall and the brain would be deprived of fuel. Result: death!

Prevention of hypoglycaemia: major concepts

1. The preferred fuel of the brain is glucose. If the blood glucose concentration falls (hypoglycaemia), the brain is deprived of fuel (neuroglycopaenia) which progressively results in unconsciousness, coma, brain damage and inevitably death.

2. The immediate reserve of glucose is liver glycogen. This is mobilised by glucagon within a few hours of fasting to maintain the normal blood glucose concentration. (NB Muscle glycogen is reserved for its own use)

3. The brain cannot use fatty acids as a fuel. This is because they are transported in the blood bound to albumin which is too big to cross the blood-brain barrier.

4. The brain uses ketone bodies as fuel. If starvation continues for more than 2 days, the brain adapts to using the ketone bodies as a fuel. Remember, during fasting, the liver converts fatty acids to ketone bodies.

5. Muscles and other tissues are converted to glucose. During starvation, tissue proteins are broken down (tissue wasting) to form amino acids. The liver metabolises the "glucogenic" amino acids by gluconeogenesis to glucose (Chapter 46). The "ketogenic" amino acids are metabolised by the liver to form the ketone bodies, while some amino acids are both ketogenic and glucogenic.

6. Fatty acids cannot form glucose. During starvation, it is most unfortunate that **fatty acids cannot be metabolised to glucose** (Chapter

32). This means that once the glycogen reserves are exhausted, the principal gluconeogenic precursors are amino acids which are derived from tissue breakdown.

The harmful effects of hyperglycaemia

In uncontrolled diabetes mellitus, the blood glucose concentration commonly rises to 20 mMol/l (hyperglycaemia) but, in extreme cases, blood glucose concentrations of up to 60 mMol/l are seen. Although glucose is an important metabolic fuel, an abnormally high blood glucose concentration is harmful for the following reasons.

1. Osmotic effect. High blood glucose concentrations significantly increase the osmotic pressure of the blood resulting in water diffusing from the cells, into the blood and being excreted by the kidneys. The result is that the tissues become dehydrated, and dehydration of the brain cells inevitably results in coma.

2. Protein glycation. Modest increases in the blood glucose concentration result in glucose reacting non-enzymically with the free amino groups of amino acid residues in cellular and extracellular proteins. They are associated with the development in the chronic complications associated with diabetes such as neuropathy, nephropathy and retinopathy, see Chapter 33.

3. Formation of reactive oxygen species (ROS). Evidence suggests that hyperglycaemia results in the formation of ROS (Chapter 19). Because ROS damage lipids, protein and DNA, they are thought to contribute to the pathogenesis of diabetic complications.

The five phases of glucose homeostasis

Figure 25.1 illustrates the origin of blood glucose following a meal and then progressing to a 40-day fast. The origin of the blood glucose can be classified into five phases.

1. Absorptive phase I. When dietary (exogenous) carbohydrate is digested and absorbed, glucose is abundant and the blood glucose concentration tends to rise. Insulin is secreted from pancreatic β-cells. Liver and muscle metabolise glucose to glycogen. When the glycogen reserves are full, liver metabolises glucose to triacylglycerols which are transported as VLDL to the adipose tissue for storage.

2. Post-absorptive phase II. After about 3 hours, the exogenous glucose will have been disposed of. The pancreatic α-cells secrete glucagon and this promotes the breakdown of liver glycogen, which contributes to the blood glucose concentration. Note that after about 6 hours, glucagon begins to stimulate the liver to perform gluconeogenesis.

3. Early starvation phase III. Approximately 14 hours after the meal (which approximates to the interval between an early evening dinner and a leisurely breakfast) the glucose being used is derived equally from glycogen and gluconeogenesis. Glucose derived from glycogen continues to decline whereas glucose derived from gluconeogenesis becomes more important until 32 hours of starvation.

4. Intermediate starvation phase IV. After 32 hours of starvation, the liver's glycogen reserves are exhausted. From now on, the only source of glucose is gluconeogenesis which is produced under the influence of the glucocorticosteroid hormone, cortisol. Fortunately, since gluconeogenesis is associated with tissue wasting, the liver produces ketone bodies from fatty acids and the brain adapts to use ketone bodies as a fuel. This process spares glucose and helps to minimise the provision of gluconeogenic substrates by muscle wasting.

5. Prolonged starvation phase V. After about 16 days starvation, an average person with access to water might survive another 24 days without food in phase V of glucose homeostasis (i.e. a total of 40 days). During this final phase, glucose is provided entirely by gluconeogenesis. The ketone bodies are now the major fuel of the brain, thereby sparing glucose which is consumed by the brain at a diminished rate.

Gluconeogenesis, muscle wasting and failure of wound healing

Although glucagon begins to stimulate gluconeogenesis after about 6 hours of fasting, it is from 32 hours onwards when cortisol contributes to gluconeogenesis that it is maximally stimulated. *NB The glucocorticosteroid hormone* **cortisol** *is a catabolic steroid and is active in the breakdown of proteins in muscle and other tissues to form amino acids which are used as gluconeogenic precursors*. Obviously, muscle wasting is a desperate strategy to supply the brain with glucose for energy metabolism. This observation leads to the importance of nutritional support in patients who are recovering from surgery or major injury such as crush syndrome or severe burns. If the patient is not consuming sufficient food, then a catabolic state will prevail. The result is that muscle and tissue wasting will occur, contrary to the need for the patient to be in an anabolic state enabling repair of the wounds.

Glucose-stimulated secretion of insulin from β-cells

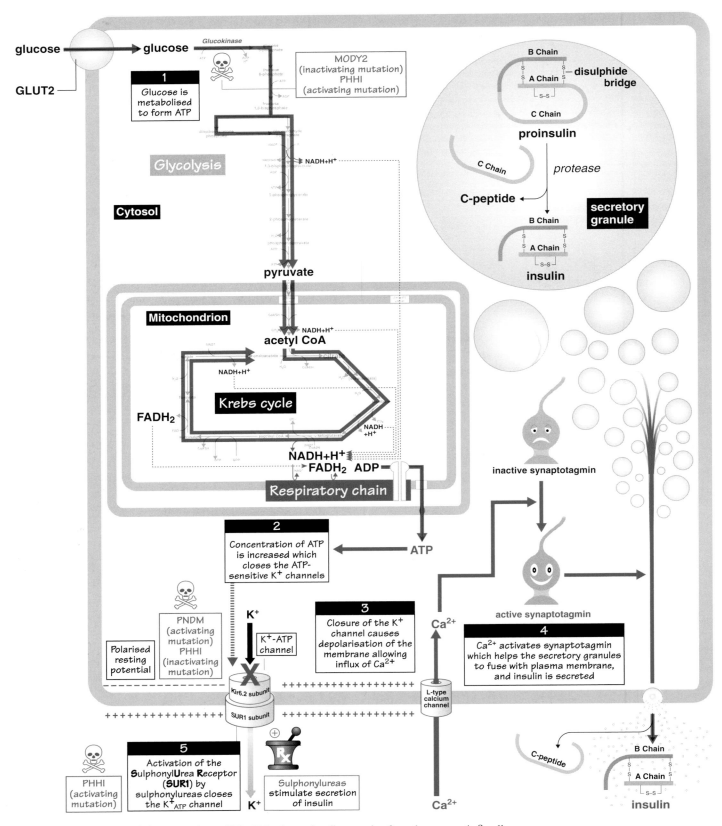

Figure 26.1 Metabolism of glucose produces ATP which triggers insulin secretion from the pancreatic β-cell.

Table 26.1 Metabolism of glucose produces ATP which triggers insulin secretion from the pancreatic β-cell, see Fig. 26.1.

1 Glucose enters the β-cell via the **GLUT2** glucose transporter and is phosphorylated by **glucokinase** prior to being metabolised by **glycolysis**, **Krebs cycle** and the **respiratory chain** to produce **ATP**

2 When the concentration of ATP increases, it **closes** the **ATP-sensitive potassium channels** (K_{ATP} channels)

3 At rest, the plasma membrane is polarised. It has a resting potential with the inside of the membrane having a negative charge. When the **potassium channels are closed by ATP, K^+ ions (positively charged) accumulate and** neutralise the negative charges on the inside surface of the membrane thus **depolarising the membrane.** Depolarisation activates calcium channels causing an **influx of Ca^{2+} ions**

4 Ca^{2+} ions **activate synaptotagmin** which helps the secretory granules containing insulin to fuse with the plasma membrane and insulin is secreted

5 **Kir6.2/SUR1 complex.** The **sulphonylurea** drugs (e.g. glibenclamide, gliclazide, tolbutamide) bind to **SUR1** (**s**ulphony**l**urea **r**eceptor) causing it to close the K_{ATP} channels (Kir6.2) which depolarises **the membrane and promotes insulin secretion**

β-cell metabolism

The β-cells are the cells within the islets of Langerhans of the pancreas that manufacture, store and secrete insulin. Insulin is secreted after a meal and the metabolic fuel hypothesis proposes this is linked to the metabolism of glucose by the β-cells to produce ATP, and ATP is the biochemical signal that triggers insulin secretion. Thus, when increasing amounts of carbohydrate-containing food are absorbed, then increasing amounts of glucose will be metabolised to ATP and this will trigger proportionate amounts of insulin to be secreted.

The several steps in this process are summarised in Table 26.1 (relating to Fig. 26.1).

Inborn errors of β-cell metabolism can cause excessive or insufficient production of insulin

These are rare inborn errors which result in **hypo**glycaemia or **hyper**glycaemia, respectively.

Excessive production of insulin

Inappropriate hypersecretion of insulin causes **p**ersistent **h**yperinsulinaemic **h**ypoglycaemia of **i**nfancy (**PHHI**). PHHI occurs in patients with an activating mutation in the glucokinase (GCK) gene. PHHI also occurs when there is an inactivating mutation of the potassium channel, Kir6.2 (Table 26.2, Fig. 26.1).

Insufficient production of insulin

Maturity **o**nset **d**iabetes of the **y**oung (**MODY**) is usually a mild form of diabetes which results from an inactivating mutation of the gene coding glucokinase or the transcription factors regulating insulin synthesis and secretion.

The onset of **p**ermanent **n**eonatal **d**iabetes **m**ellitus (**PNDM**) is usually within 6 months of birth and hitherto patients have been treated with insulin for life. However, recently it has been shown that about 30% of these babies have an activating mutation in the gene encoding the Kir6.2 subunit of the K_{ATP} potassium channels*. These mutations result in insufficient production of insulin and consequently PNDM (Table 26.2, Fig. 26.1). However, if the diagnosis is confirmed by genetic testing, they may be treated with sulphonylureas.

Structure of the insulin molecule

Proinsulin is stored in the β-cells. It is converted to insulin in the secretory granules by proteases. Proteolytic cleavage of the C-chain produces active insulin, i.e. a dimer of the A- and B-chains.

Table 26.2 Inborn errors of β-cell metabolism.

Glucokinase: heterozygous, activating mutation	**Glucokinase** is **hyperactive** causing inappropriately high β-cell glucose metabolism resulting in excessive insulin secretion and **p**ersistent **h**yperinsulinaemic **h**ypoglycaemia of infancy (**PHHI**)
Glucokinase: heterozygous, inactivating mutation	**Glucokinase** is **less active** causing decreased β-cell glucose metabolism resulting in decreased insulin secretion and **m**aturity **o**nset **d**iabetes of the **y**oung (**MODY 2**)
Kir6.2: heterozygous, activating mutation (**K** inwardly **r**ectifying channel)	K_{ATP} channels are **constantly active** (open) which prevents insulin secretion and causes **p**ermanent **n**eonatal **d**iabetes **m**ellitus (**PNDM**). Recent studies show these patients (who previously were given insulin) respond to sulphonylurea therapy
Kir6.2: heterozygous, inactivating mutation	K_{ATP} channels are **constantly inactive** (closed) which triggers constant insulin secretion causing **p**ersistent **h**yperinsulinaemic **h**ypoglycaemia of infancy (**PHHI**)
SUR1: heterozygous, activating mutation (**s**ulphony**l**urea **r**eceptor)	The **active** SUR1 mutation constantly stimulates closure of the K_{ATP} channel causing constant insulin secretion and **PHHI**
An inactivating mutation has not been described	

*Gloyn AL, Pearson ER, Antcliff JF et al. (2004) Activating mutations in the gene encoding the ATP-sensitive potassium-channel subunit Kir 6.2 and permanent neonatal diabetes. N Eng J Med **350**, 1838–49.

27 Regulation of glycogen metabolism

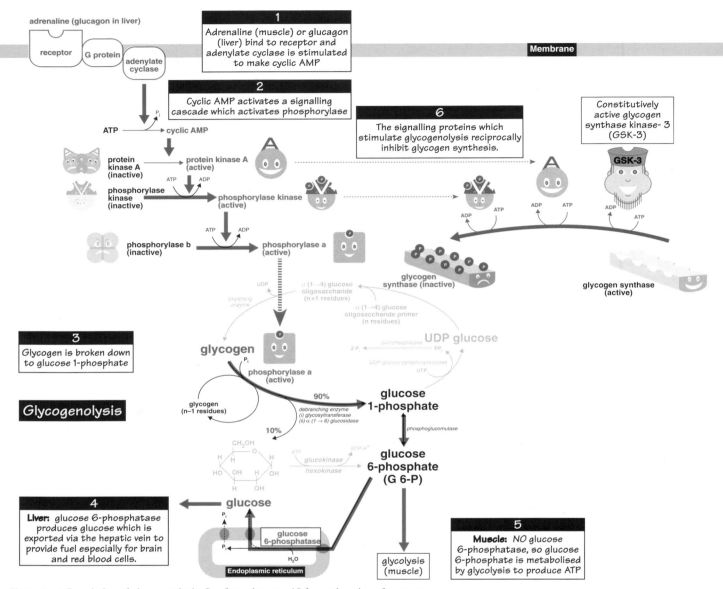

1
Adrenaline (muscle) or glucagon (liver) bind to receptor and adenylate cyclase is stimulated to make cyclic AMP

2
Cyclic AMP activates a signalling cascade which activates phosphorylase

6
The signalling proteins which stimulate glycogenolysis reciprocally inhibit glycogen synthesis.

Constitutively active glycogen synthase kinase- 3 (GSK-3)

adrenaline (glucagon in liver)

receptor   G protein

adenylate cyclase

Membrane

ATP → cyclic AMP

protein kinase A (inactive) → protein kinase A (active)

phosphorylase kinase (inactive) → phosphorylase kinase (active)

phosphorylase b (inactive) → phosphorylase a (active)

GSK-3

glycogen synthase (inactive)   glycogen synthase (active)

UDP

α (1→4) glucose oligosaccharide (n+1 residues)

α (1→4) glucose oligosaccharide primer (n residues)

branching enzyme

3
Glycogen is broken down to glucose 1-phosphate

Glycogenolysis

glycogen

phosphorylase a (active)

glycogen (n−1 residues)

UDP glucose

2 Pᵢ   PP

UDP glucose pyrophosphorylase   UTP

90% → **glucose 1-phosphate**

10%

debranching enzyme
(i) glycosyltransferase
(ii) α (1 → 6) glucosidase

phosphoglucomutase

CH₂OH

glucokinase
hexokinase

glucose 6-phosphate (G 6-P)

4
Liver: glucose 6-phosphatase produces glucose which is exported via the hepatic vein to provide fuel especially for brain and red blood cells.

glucose

glucose 6-phosphatase

H₂O

Endoplasmic reticulum

glycolysis (muscle)

5
Muscle: NO glucose 6-phosphatase, so glucose 6-phosphate is metabolised by glycolysis to produce ATP

Figure 27.1 Regulation of glycogenolysis. See figure key on p10 for explanation of cartoons.

Regulation of glycogenolysis

Glycogen is stored mainly in liver and muscle. The **liver** (the great provider) breaks down glycogen during periods of fasting to top-up the blood glucose concentration for use as fuel by the brain and red blood cells. On the other hand, **muscle** (the fuel guzzler) uses glycogen for its own energy needs, especially for anaerobic glycolysis in a "flight or fight" emergency. In **muscle**, **adrenaline** initiates glycogenolysis by binding to its receptor and stimulating **adenylate cyclase** to produce **cyclic AMP**. Cyclic AMP activates a cascade of reactions which finally activates **phosphorylase** causing glycogen breakdown. In the **liver**, **glucagon**, which is released from pancreatic α-cells during fasting, initiates glycogenolysis.

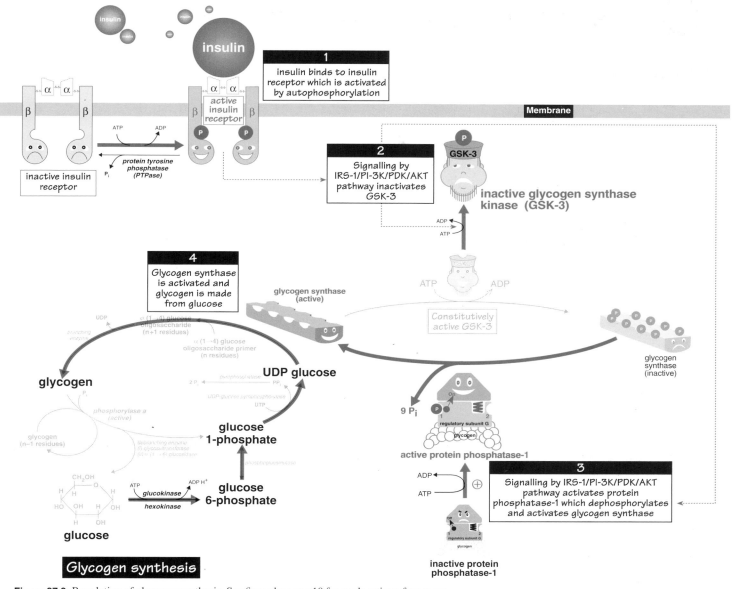

Figure 27.2 Regulation of glycogen synthesis. See figure key on p10 for explanation of cartoons.

Regulation of glycogen synthesis

Glycogen synthesis is initiated when **insulin** binds to its **receptor**. This causes autophosphorylation of tyrosine residues in the insulin receptor which triggers a chain of signalling proteins (**IRS-1/PI-3 kinase/PDK/AKT** Chapter 29); which inactivates **glycogen synthase kinase-3 (GSK-3)**. During **fasting**, GSK-3 is constitutively **active**. In other words, it is only **inactive** after **feeding** in response to insulin signalling. As such, when fasting, **active GSK-3** applies the brakes to glycogen synthesis by phosphorylating and thus inactivating **glycogen synthase**. When insulin renders **GSK-3 inactive**, the signalling pathway **activates protein phosphatase-1** which dephosphorylates and **activates**

glycogen synthase. Glycogen synthesis from glucose can now proceed.

Protein tyrosine phosphatase (PTPase) and PTPase inhibitors

Once feeding is finished, the insulin signal is terminated by dephosphorylating the tyrosine residues of the insulin receptor using PTPase. In a subgroup of type 2 diabetic patients, PTPase is inappropriately active which results in attenuation of the insulin signal causing insulin resistance. Current research to discover PTPase inhibitors promises a novel treatment for type 2 diabetes.

Glycogen breakdown (glycogenolysis) and glycogen storage diseases

Glycogenolysis in health

Glycogen is stored in muscle and liver. It is mobilised in liver during starvation and in muscle during extreme exercise.

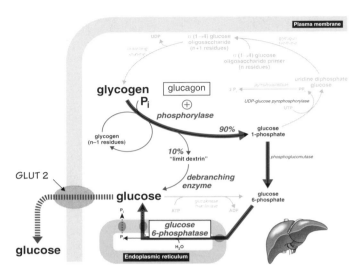

Figure 28.1 Normal glycogenolysis in liver. Liver is the great provider and during fasting (when glucagon prevails) its reserves of glycogen are broken down to release glucose in to the blood where it is transported to the brain for energy metabolism. To achieve this, **liver has glucose 6-phosphatase activity**.

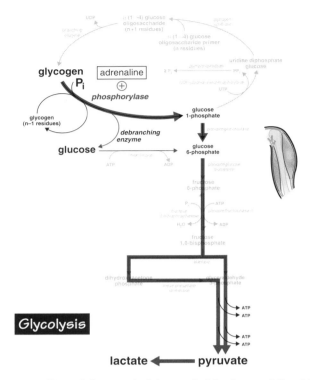

Figure 28.2 Normal glycogenolysis in muscle. Muscle, especially white skeletal muscle, uses glycogen entirely for its own benefit as a fuel during vigorous anaerobic exercise, e.g. during adrenaline-stimulated flight or fight. **Muscle does not have glucose 6-phosphatase activity.**

Glycogen storage diseases (GSD)

The twelve glycogen storage diseases are characterised by abnormal accumulation of glycogen. Four examples are shown (Figs 28.3–28.6).

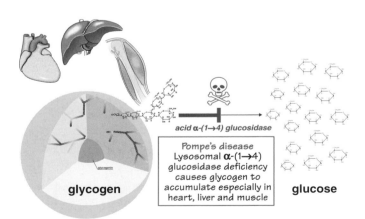

Figure 28.3 GSD II, Pompe's disease. GSD II (autosomal recessive) is caused by a deficiency of acid α-(1 → 4) glucosidase, a lysosomal enzyme. Glycogen accumulates causing cardiomegaly after 2–3 months. The liver and muscle are also affected causing generalised muscle weakness. GSD II is a target for enzyme replacement therapy.

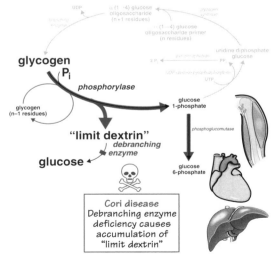

Figure 28.4 GSD III, Cori disease. This is named after husband and wife, Carl and Gerty Cori (so note the apostrophe if you prefer "Coris's" disease). GSD III is caused by a deficiency of **debranching enzyme** so **"limit dextrin"** accumulates which is an abnormal form of glycogen where the branches are reduced to α-(1 → 6) stumps. GSD III presents with hypoglycaemia and hepatomegaly.

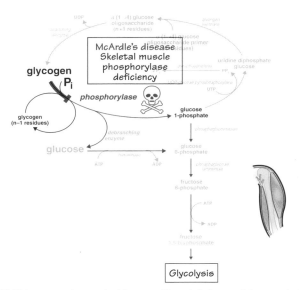

Figure 28.5 GSD V, McArdle's disease. GSD V (autosomal recessive) is caused by a deficiency of the muscle form of **phosphorylase** (myophosphorylase). Consequently, GSD III patients are unable to mobilise glycogen for energy metabolism, which results in fatigue, muscle pain and myoglobinuria following exercise.

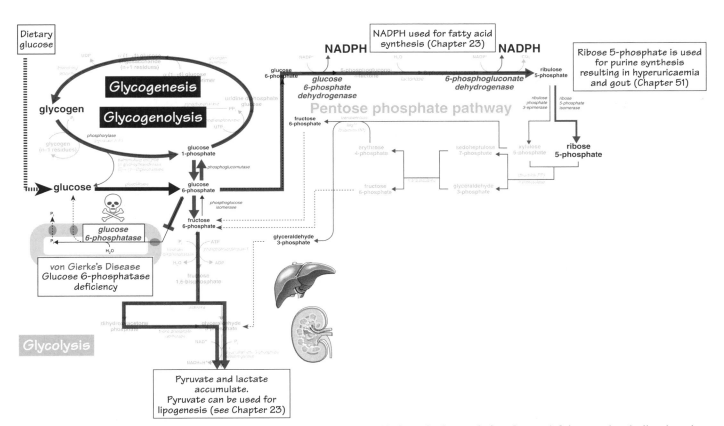

Figure 28.6 GSD I, von Gierke's disease. GSD I (autosomal recessive) is caused by **hepatic glucose 6-phosphatase** deficiency and so the liver loses its ability to prevent hypoglycaemia. Neonatal hypoglycaemia can be severe and glycogen is stored in excess in the liver and kidney. Other features that are a consequence of accumulation of glucose 6-phosphate are: hyperlactataemia, hyperlipidaemia, hyperuricaemia and gout.

29 Insulin signal transduction and diabetes mellitus

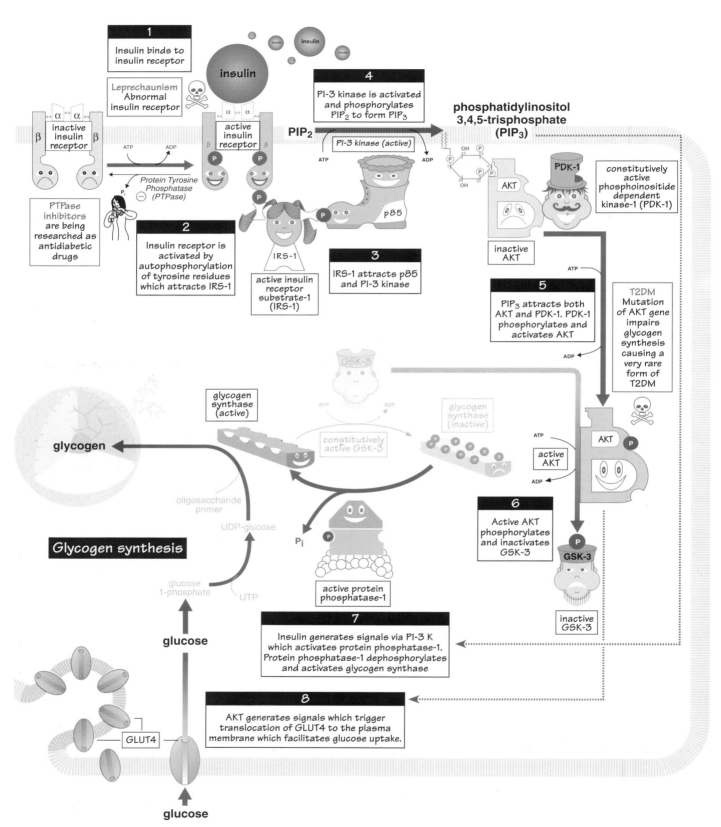

Figure 29.1 How insulin signal transduction stimulates glycogen synthesis (PDK/AKT hypothesis). See figure key on p.10 for explanation of cartoons.

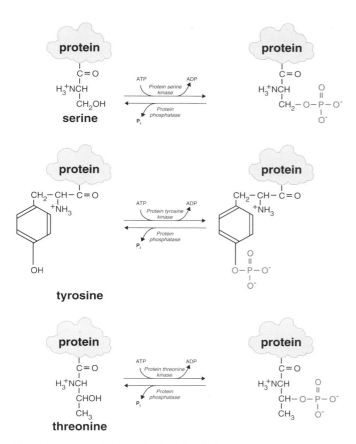

Figure 29.2 Reversible protein phosphorylation.

Regulation of enzyme activity by reversible protein phosphorylation

Approximately one-third of cellular proteins contain phosphate and are subject to covalent modification by **phosphorylation** and **dephosphorylation** reactions. This reversible phosphorylation of proteins causes conformational changes in the protein which dramatically alters their properties, e.g. from an active to an inactive enzyme, or *vice versa*. The sites of protein phosphorylation are those amino acid residues that contain hydroxyl groups, most commonly **serine** but also **tyrosine** and **threonine**, (Fig. 29.2, Chapter 10). Phosphorylation is by **protein kinase** and dephosphorylation is by **protein phosphatase**. The importance of reversible protein phosphorylation to the living cell is emphasised by the fact that protein kinases and protein phosphatases comprise approximately 5% of the proteins encoded by the human genome. Current research is discovering abnormalities of protein phosphorylation that are associated with diseases, notably **t**ype 2 **d**iabetes **m**ellitus (T2DM) and cancer. In the future, the discovery of drugs that modify protein phosphorylation/dephosphorylation promises new therapies for the treatment of these diseases.

Insulin signal transduction: The PDK/AKT hypothesis

AKT was previously known as PKB. Insulin has scores of different effects on cells. It can stimulate the translocation of GLUT4 glucose transporters to the plasma membrane, and stimulate fatty acid synthesis, protein synthesis, glycogen synthesis, etc. Remarkably all these effects are mediated though one insulin receptor and this phenomenon is known as the **pleiotropic** effects of insulin (pleiotropic is from the Greek meaning, "many ways"). The process begins with the binding of insulin to its receptor, which initiates a series of interactions between various signalling protein eventually resulting in an event which stimulates or inhibits a regulatory process.

In Fig. 29.1, we see how insulin binds to the insulin receptor. This activates tyrosine residues on the insulin receptor by the process of **autophosphorylation**. Once the insulin receptor is activated, it attracts and binds **insulin receptor substrate-1 (IRS-1)**. IRS-1 now attracts **p85** which is the regulatory subunit of PI-3 **kinase**. PI-3 kinase phosphorylates the 3 position of **phosphatidylinositol 4,5-bisphosphate (PIP₂)** to form **phosphatidylinositol 3,4,5-trisphosphate (PIP₃)**. PIP₃ now attracts to the membrane **AKT** (previously known as **PKB**) and **PDK-1** so they are adjacent and **AKT** is activated by phosphorylation. AKT can now phosphorylate and inactivate **glycogen synthase kinase-3 (GSK-3)**. GSK-3 is constitutively active and in the fasting state (i.e. in the absence of insulin), it phosphorylates and **inactivates glycogen synthase** which applies the brakes to the process of glycogen synthesis. So, we have now seen how insulin through AKT removes the inhibition by GSK-3 and **glycogen synthase is activated** following dephosphorylation by **protein phosphatase-1**. Meanwhile, another chain of signals mediated by AKT stimulates the translocation of **GLUT4** glucose transporters to the plasma membrane which facilitates glucose uptake. The glucose can be metabolised to glycogen in the presence of active glycogen synthase.

Disorders of insulin signal transduction

Recent clinical research provides support for the validity of the PDK/AKT hypothesis and three examples are shown below.

Leprechaunism (Donohue syndrome)

This is a very rare inborn error in which babies fail to thrive and have the features of mythical Irish elves know as "leprechauns". This causes severe diabetes and premature death. The insulin receptor is abnormal and cannot function adequately. This results in a failure of insulin signalling even though the β-cells of the pancreas are able to secrete insulin.

AKT (or PKB) mutation

Recently, a family has been described with a mutation of the gene that expresses AKT[*]. As predicted by the PDK/AKT hypothesis, this results in a very rare form of type 2 diabetes.

Protein tyrosine phosphatase

When feeding has finished, insulin secretion stops and insulin signal transduction within the cell must be terminated. Dephosphorylation of the insulin receptor by **protein tyrosine phosphatase (PTPase)** occurs which inactivates the insulin receptor and insulin signalling ceases. However, there is evidence that some diabetic patients have a form of PTPase that is inappropriately active and opposes normal activation of the receptor by phosphorylation. Currently, there is a major research effort to develop drugs that inhibit PTPase and provide a new treatment for type 2 diabetes.

[*] George S, Rochford JJ, Wolfrum C *et al.* (2004) A family with severe insulin resistance and diabetes due to mutation in AKT2. *Science* **304**, 1325–8.

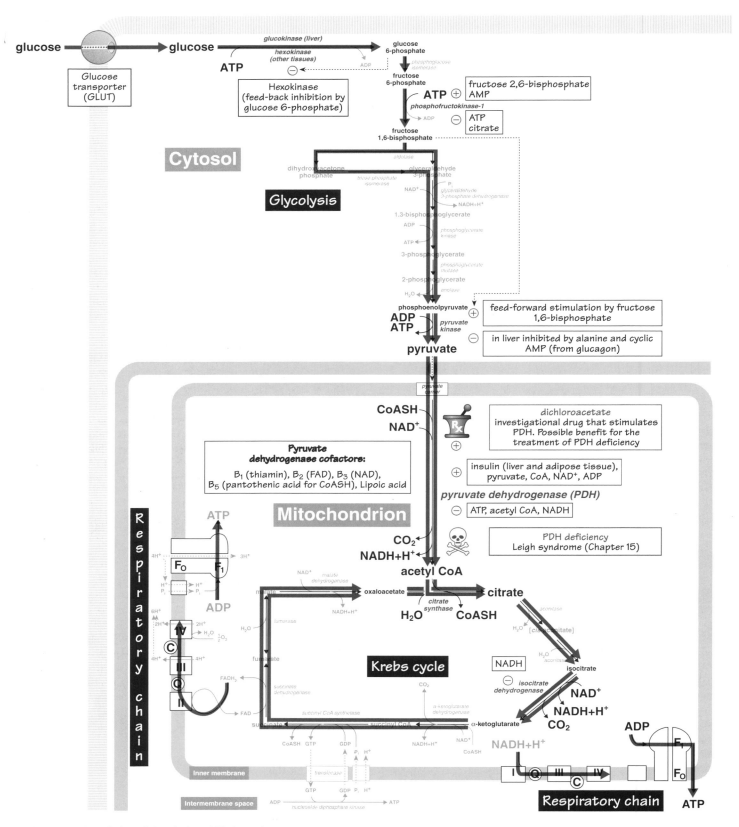

Figure 30.1 Regulation of glycolysis and Krebs cycle.

Regulation of glycolysis

Glycolysis has different functions in different tissues. In **anaerobic** tissues such as white muscle, retina and in red blood cells, its main function is the production of ATP with lactate the end product (Chapter 21). Under **aerobic** conditions in muscle, glycolysis provides pyruvate for oxidation in Krebs cycle which cooperates with the respiratory chain to make ATP. In liver and adipose tissue, glycolysis, co-operates with the pentose phosphate pathway to produce pyruvate for fatty acid synthesis. *NB Nature has good reasons for its design of metabolic regulation! When studying metabolic pathways, remember that the regulation of metabolism is directed to their functions.*

Glycolysis is regulated by: (i) **glucose transporters (GLUTs)**, (ii) **glucokinase** or **hexokinase**, (iii) **phosphofructokinase-1**, (iv) **pyruvate kinase**, and (v) **pyruvate dehydrogenase**.

Glucose transporters (GLUTs)

Glucose enters a cell via **glucose transporters (GLUTs)**. There are several types, e.g. **GLUT1, GLUT2**, etc. Glucose transporters are located in the plasma membrane except for **GLUT4**, which controls glycolysis in **muscle** and **adipose tissue**. During fasting, **GLUT4** transporters are located in intracellular vesicles. After feeding, **insulin** causes the vesicles to recruit the GLUT4s into the plasma membrane enabling glucose transport into the cell.

Glucokinase and hexokinase

The first reaction of glycolysis is the phosphorylation of glucose to glucose 6-phosphate catalysed by hexokinase or glucokinase. **Hexokinase** is found in most types of cell and has a low Km (i.e. a high affinity) for glucose, and is subject to feedback inhibition by **glucose 6-phosphate**. **Glucokinase** has a high Km (i.e. low affinity) for glucose and is found in liver and the β-cells of pancreas. In liver, it is well adapted to cope with the high concentrations of glucose (up to 15 mMol/l) transported from the intestines by the hepatic portal vein after a carbohydrate meal. *(Remember: gLucokinase is found in the Liver.)*

Phosphofructokinase-1 (PFK-1)

Stimulation of PFK-1 PFK-1 is stimulated by **fructose 2,6-bisphosphate (F 2,6-bisP)**. PFK-1 is also stimulated by **AMP** which, when abundant, indicates a **low** energy state and the need for ATP synthesis requiring increased glycolysis.

*(Production of F 2,6-bisP is **stimulated** by insulin in liver, and by high fructose 6-phosphate concentrations in skeletal muscle. F 2,6-bisP is **depleted** by glucagon in liver, and by low fructose 6-phosphate concentrations in skeletal muscle.)*

Inhibition of PFK-1: When **ATP** is abundant, it inhibits PFK-1 and restricts glycolysis. Another inhibitor of PFK-1 is **citrate**.

Pyruvate kinase (PK)

Inhibition of PK In **liver**, pyruvate kinase is **inhibited** by **alanine** and **cyclic AMP** (which is produced under the influence of **glucagon**). Glucagon is present during fasting, as is the gluconeogenic precursor alanine, which is derived from muscle protein (Chapter 44). Inhibition of PK restricts phosphoenolpyruvate catabolism and favours gluconeogenesis (Chapter 46).

Stimulation of PK In **liver**, pyruvate kinase is **stimulated** by **fructose 1,6-bisphosphate** (feed-forward stimulation). This is especially important during the transition from fasting (gluconeogenesis, PK inhibited) to lipogenesis (PK active) (Chapter 23).

Pyruvate dehydrogenase (PDH)

PDH is a complex of three enzymes located in the mitochondrion, which controls the rate of entry of pyruvate into Krebs cycle.

Stimulation of PDH After a carbohydrate meal, PDH is **stimulated** by **insulin** in liver and adipose tissue where pyruvate is destined for fatty acid synthesis (Chapter 23). PDH is also stimulated by its substrate **pyruvate**, and by the availability of its coenzymes **CoA**, and **NAD⁺**. Finally, PDH is stimulated by **ADP** which is increased in the low-energy state and indicates the need for ATP synthesis by cooperation of Krebs cycle and the respiratory chain.

Inhibition of PDH PDH is inhibited by **ATP** when it is abundant thereby restricting the oxidation of pyruvate by Krebs cycle. PDH is also inhibited by **acetyl CoA** and **NADH**, which are products of the PDH reaction. Since acetyl CoA and NADH are also abundant fatty acids are used as metabolic fuel and their inhibition of pyruvate dehydrogenase helps to conserves pyruvate (NB during starvation, pyruvate is made from food reserves, e.g. glycogen and amino acids derived from muscle protein (Chapter 46)).

Regulation of Krebs cycle

Krebs cycle has different functions in different tissues. For example, in **muscle** and **brain** it oxidises acetylCoA to form NADH and FADH₂ which are used to generate ATP in the respiratory chain (Chapters 15–17). In **liver**, **during fasting**, acetyl CoA is not oxidised by Krebs cycle. Instead, sections of Krebs cycle operate to direct amino acid derivates towards malate for gluconeogenesis (Chapter 46). In **liver and adipose tissue**, **after feeding**, the destiny of acetyl CoA is a brief sojourn in Krebs cycle by incorporation into citrate before export to the cytosol for biosynthesis to fatty acids (Chapter 23).

Isocitrate dehydrogenase (ICDH)

Isocitrate dehydrogenase is inhibited when NADH accumulates. This is obvious when it realised that the coenzyme for ICDH is NAD⁺, which is depleted when it has been reduced to NADH.

Disorders of PDH activity
Thiamin deficiency

Nerve tissue is mainly dependent for ATP production on glucose metabolism via glycolysis to produce acetyl CoA by the PDH reaction for oxidation in Krebs cycle. Since thiamin is essential for PDH activity, thiamin deficiency, which can occur in malnourished alcoholics, results in PDH dysfunction and an energy deficit in nerve tissue. This causes hyperlactataemia and neuropathy which can progress to Wernicke's encephalopathy and Korsakoff's psychosis (Chapter 55).

(Remember that although fatty acids produce acetyl CoA independently of PDH, they are not available to the brain for fuel as they cannot cross the blood-brain barrier.)

Leigh syndrome

Some forms of Leigh syndrome are caused by PDH dysfunction (Chapter 15).

31 Oxidation of fatty acids to produce ATP in muscle and ketone bodies in liver

Yield of ATP from the complete oxidation of palmitate		
Reaction	NADH or FADH$_2$	ATP yield
1 Long-chain acyl CoA synthetase		–2
2 Acyl CoA dehydrogenase (× 7)	7 FADH$_2$	10.5
3 L-3-hydroxyacyl CoA dehydrogenase (× 7)	7 NADH	17.5
4 Isocitrate dehydrogenase	8 NADH	20
5 α-Ketoglutarate dehydrogenase	8 NADH	20
6 Succinyl CoA synthetase/nucleoside diphosphate kinase		8
7 Succinate dehydrogenase	8 FADH$_2$	12
8 Malate dehydrogenase	8 NADH	20
	TOTAL	106

NB The total of 106 does not allow for the energy used to transport phosphate (equivalent to 2 ATPs) so true net yield is 104 ATP, see JG Salway, Metabolism at a Glance, 3rd ed pp 38—39, Blackwell Publishing

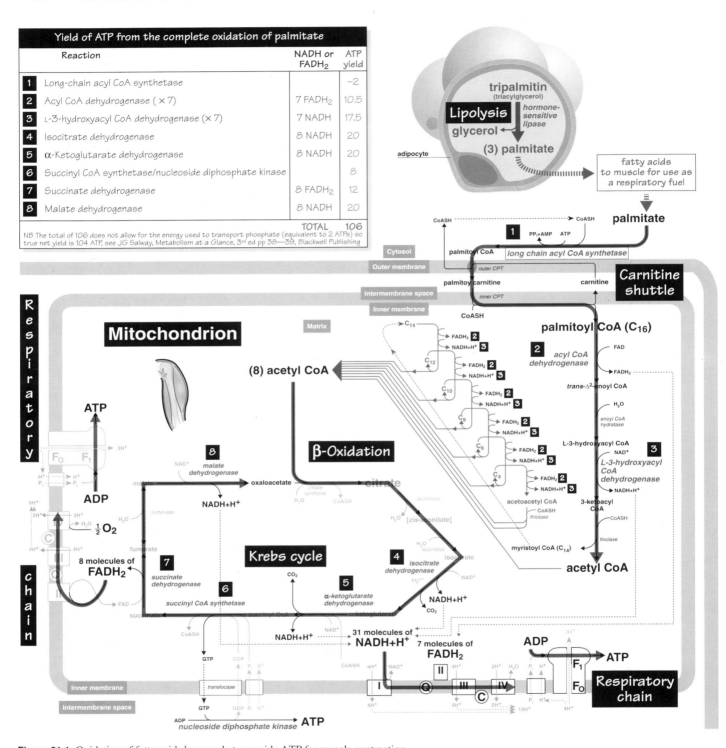

Figure 31.1 Oxidation of fatty acids by muscle to provide ATP for muscle contraction.

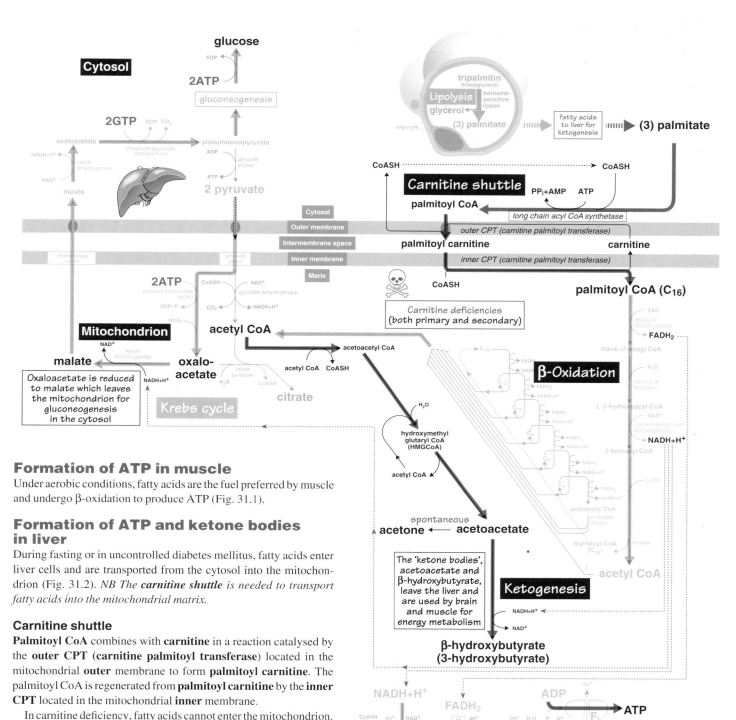

Figure 31.2 Oxidation of fatty acids by liver to provide ATP for gluconeogenesis and acetyl CoA for ketogenesis.

Formation of ATP in muscle

Under aerobic conditions, fatty acids are the fuel preferred by muscle and undergo β-oxidation to produce ATP (Fig. 31.1).

Formation of ATP and ketone bodies in liver

During fasting or in uncontrolled diabetes mellitus, fatty acids enter liver cells and are transported from the cytosol into the mitochondrion (Fig. 31.2). *NB The **carnitine shuttle** is needed to transport fatty acids into the mitochondrial matrix.*

Carnitine shuttle

Palmitoyl CoA combines with **carnitine** in a reaction catalysed by the **outer CPT (carnitine palmitoyl transferase)** located in the mitochondrial **outer** membrane to form **palmitoyl carnitine**. The palmitoyl CoA is regenerated from **palmitoyl carnitine** by the **inner CPT** located in the mitochondrial **inner** membrane.

In carnitine deficiency, fatty acids cannot enter the mitochondrion. Consequently β-oxidation is inhibited resulting in hypoglycaemia.

Ketogenesis

Fatty acids undergo β-oxidation producing acetyl CoA, NADH and FADH$_2$. The NADH and FADH$_2$ are oxidised by the respiratory chain to form ATP which is used for gluconeogenesis (Chapter 32) and for urea synthesis (Chapter 44). The acetyl CoA forms the "ketone bodies" **acetoacetate** and **β-hydroxybutyrate. Acetone**, formed in small amounts from acetoacetate, causes the fruity smell of the breath in ketotic patients or people on low carbohydrate diets. NB When the ratio of NADH/NAD$^+$ is high as in **diabetic ketoacidosis (DKA)**, the equilibrium of the **β-hydroxybutyrate dehydrogenase** reaction favours β-hydroxybutyrate production. Hence acetoacetate in DKA can be 20% of the β-hydroxybutyrate concentration. **Warning**: the nitroprusside reaction used to detect "ketone bodies" measures only acetoacetate and **not** the principal ketone body, β-hydroxybutyrate.

32 Regulation of lipolysis, β-oxidation, ketogenesis and gluconeogenesis

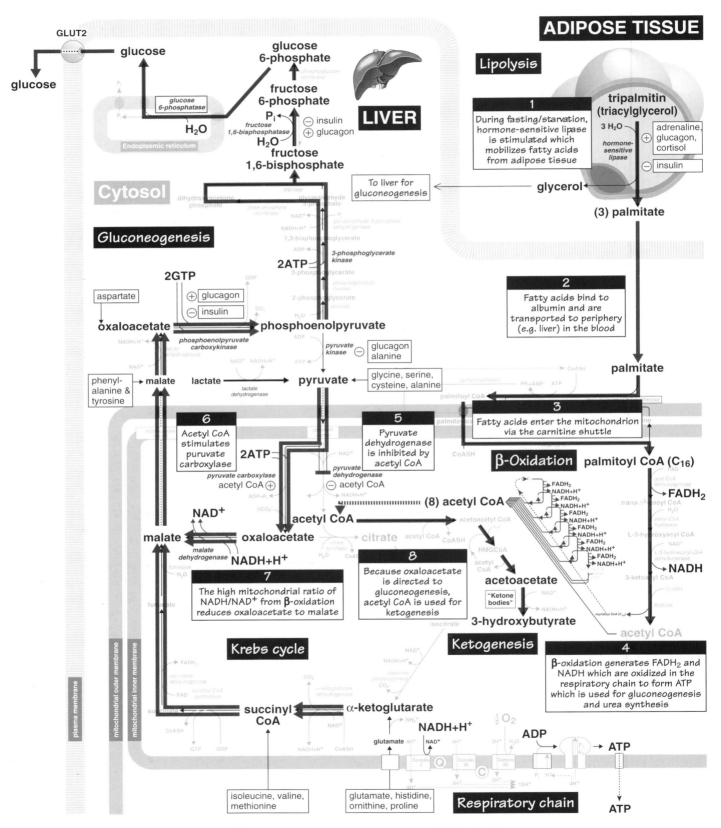

Figure 32.1 The relationship between lipolysis, β-oxidation, gluconeogenesis and ketogenesis in fasting liver.

Figure 32.1 The relationship between lipolysis, β-oxidation, gluconeogenesis, and ketogenesis in fasting liver

1 *During fasting or starvation, the catabolic hormones* **glucagon** *and* **cortisol** *are secreted from the α-cells of the pancreas and the adrenal cortex respectively. In response to severe stress or danger, adrenaline is secreted by the adrenal medulla.* **These hormones stimulate hormone-sensitive lipase which mobilizes fatty acids and glycerol from white adipose tissue**

2 *The* **fatty acids** *bind to albumin and are transported in the blood to the liver.*

3 **Fatty acids** *enter the mitochondrion via the carnitine shuttle.*

4 **β-oxidation** *of the fatty acids generates FADH$_2$ and NADH and acetylCoA. FADH$_2$ and NADH are oxidsed in the respiratory chain to supply ATP for gluconeogenesis.*

5 **Acetyl CoA** *inhibits pyravate dehydrogenase*

6 **Acetyl CoA** *stimulates pyruvate carboxylase which converts pyruvate to oxaloacetate.*

7 **β-oxidation** *ensures that the mitochondrial ratio of NADH/NAD$^+$ is high. The high proportion of NADH reduces* **oxaloacetate** *to* **malate.** *Malate is transported from the mitochondrion into the cytosol where it forms glucose by the process of* **gluconeogenesis.**

8 **Gluconeogenesis** *is the production of glucose from non-carbohydrate substrates eg amino acids. NB 6 ATP equivalents (from β-oxidation see 4) are needed to produce 1 glucose molecule*

9 **Ketogenesis mitochondrial** *oxaloacetate is depleted. Therefore, acetylCoA cannot react with oxaloacetate to form citrate for oxidation in Krebs cycle. Instead, acetylCoA reacts with itself to form* **acetoacetate and 3-hydroxybutyrate (the ketone bodies)**

The liver maintains blood glucose during starvation

The principal fuel for the brain is glucose. If brain is deprived of glucose (**neuroglycopaenia**) the result is coma. Patients with **insulinoma** produce excessive amounts of insulin resulting in hypoglycaemia, fainting or abnormal behaviour which can be misdiagnosed as epilepsy or psychiatric disease. Similarly type 1 diabetic patients are familiar with the symptoms of hypoglycaemia and the need to prevent a "hypo" by balancing their food intake with their insulin injections.

The normal fasting blood glucose concentration is maintained between 3.5 and 5.5 mMol/l. This remarkable feat of metabolic control applies despite extremes of metabolic stress; for example, during the sudden huge demand for fuel by a 100-metre sprinter (muscle glycogen is used) or the longer term, massive fuel consumption needed by a Marathon runner (triacylglycerol plus muscle and liver glycogen). Moreover, blood glucose must be maintained above 3.5 mMol/l during short-term fasting or long-term starvation over several weeks. The liver plays a vital role in glucose homeostasis (Chapter 25).

Liver glycogen

During the first few hours of fasting, **glucagon** activates glycogen breakdown in the liver (glycogenolysis) which releases glucose into the blood preventing hypoglycaemia (Chapter 28).

Fuels used when liver glycogen is exhausted

Gluconeogenesis Liver glycogen is exhausted within 24 hours. **NB THE BRAIN CANNOT USE FATTY ACIDS AS A FUEL** and **FATTY ACIDS CANNOT BE METABOLISED TO GLUCOSE.** So, within 24 hours, the carbohydrate reserve (i.e. glycogen) is exhausted. Since fatty acids from triacylglycerol cannot be used as fuel by the brain, the principal remaining brain fuel is glucose which is made from muscle protein. Desperate needs demand desperate measures! So within 24 hours of starvation, the glucocorticoid hormone cortisol directs the metabolic pathways to break down muscle (muscle wasting!) to form amino acids, some of which can be metabolised to glucose by **gluconeogenesis. NB This emphasises the importance of nutrition in patients recovering from tissue trauma whether surgical, burns or crush injury. Wound healing will be slow if the patient does not eat and is in a gluconeogenic (muscle wasting) catabolic state.**

Ketogenesis The liver makes ketone bodies from fatty acids during fasting. Fortunately, after 2 days of fasting, the brain adapts to use the ketone bodies as fuel reducing the need for glucose and therefore decreasing the need for gluconeogenesis.

Regulation of lipolysis

Lipolysis is the process by which **fatty acids** and **glycerol** are mobilised from the triacylglycerol reserves in **white adipose tissue**. The regulatory enzyme of lipolysis is **hormone-sensitive lipase** which is stimulated by the hormones secreted during fasting, namely **glucagon** and **cortisol**. In the fed state, **insulin** inhibits hormone-sensitive lipase thus favouring triacylglycerol accumulation. NB Lipolysis produces glycerol, which is a gluconeogenic substrate and is metabolised to glucose.

The fatty acids released from adipose tissue are insoluble in the aqueous environment of the blood and bind to albumin, which transports them in the blood to the periphery.

Regulation of β-oxidation

The fatty acids must be transported into the mitochondrion where β-oxidation occurs. Transport of fatty acids through the inner mitochondrial membrane involves the **carnitine shuttle** (Chapter 23). The carnitine shuttle is inhibited by **malonyl CoA** which inactivates the outer **carnitine palmitoyl transferase**. Malonyl CoA is produced when fatty acids are being synthesised during the fed state and by inhibiting the carnitine shuttle it prevents the futile destruction by β-oxidation of the brand-new fatty acids as they are formed.

Regulation of gluconeogenesis

The regulatory enzymes of gluconeogenesis are confined to liver and the kidney.

1. Pyruvate carboxylase in the mitochondrion needs ATP and biotin, is induced by cortisol and is stimulated by acetyl CoA.

2. Phosphoenolpyruvate carboxykinase (PEPCK) in the cytosol needs GTP, is stimulated by glucagon and inhibited by insulin.

3. Fructose 1,6-bisphosphatase (F 1,6-bisP) in the cytosol is inhibited by **fructose 2,6-bisphosphate**. Fructose 2,6-bisphosphate is destroyed under the influence of glucagon. Conversely, it is synthesised under the influence of insulin.

4. Glucose 6-phosphatase is in the endoplasmic reticulum.

Regulation of ketogenesis

The rate of ketogenesis increases in proportion to the blood fatty acid concentration. It increases during fasting and especially in uncontrolled type 1 diabetes (**diabetic ketoacidosis (DKA)**).

33 Diabetes mellitus

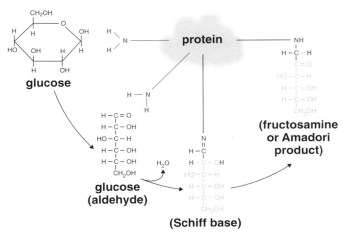

Figure 33.1 Glucose reacts non-enzymatically with free N-terminal α-amino groups and the ε-amino group of lysyl residues of proteins to form fructosamine products.

The term "diabetes" from the Greek *dia* "through" and *bainen* "to go" means "passing through" or "siphon" and describes the excessive production of urine (polyuria) in this condition. **Diabetes mellitus** (*mellitus* means "honey") refers to the sweet taste of the urine, while in diabetes insipidus the urine is "insipid" (i.e. tasteless). (Don't worry you don't have to taste the urine nowadays!) Diabetes is caused by **lack of insulin activity** while **diabetes insipidus** is caused by **insufficient vasopressin (antidiuretic hormone) activity**.

Diabetes mellitus (DM) is characterised by hyperglycaemia due to defective insulin secretion, defective insulin action or both. The global prevalence in 2004 is 150 million cases and this is projected to be 220 million in 2010. The main types are **type 1 DM** (T1DM) and **type 2 DM** (T2DM). There is also **gestational DM** and other unusual types such as **maturity onset diabetes of the young (MODY)**.

Type 1 diabetes mellitus

T1DM was previously known as "insulin dependent diabetes mellitus, (IDDM)" and "Juvenile onset diabetes (JOD)". It occurs in 0.5% of the population, and is characterised by sudden onset, usually before 25 years of age, and weight loss. The β-cells are destroyed by autoimmune attack following viral infection. "Molecular mimicry" is thought to be the cause. This happens when parts of a virus protein resemble a protein in the host's β-cells. The body's immune defences then attack **both** the **virus** and the **β-cells** which are destroyed: hence **insulin secretion ceases** causing T1DM.

Type 2 diabetes mellitus

T2DM was previously known as "non-insulin dependent diabetes mellitus (NIDDM)" and "maturity onset diabetes (MOD)". It occurs in 3–5% of the population, and is characterised by slow, insidious and progressive onset until diagnosis in middle age. T2DM is often associated with obesity.

In T2DM, insulin is present in the blood sometimes (surprisingly) at supranormal concentrations. The problem is that **although insulin is present it does not work effectively** (known as "insulin resistance").

There are probably scores of explanations why the insulin does not function, hence recent research suggests there are scores of different subtypes of T2DM. For example, insulin resistance could be caused by **structural abnormalities of any of the following**: the insulin molecule, the insulin receptor on the target tissue, the signalling proteins and enzymes involved in glucose and lipid uptake and metabolism (e.g. Chapters 23, 27, 29).

Gestational diabetes mellitus (GDM)

During pregnancy a transient period of insulin resistance is normal but in about 4% of pregnancies insulin resistance is sufficiently severe to cause hyperglycaemia and GDM ensues. The cause of insulin resistance is not clear. However, **raised** levels of **oestrogen**, **human placental lactogen**, and recently **low** levels of the insulin-sensitizer, **adiponectin**, have been implicated.

Maturity onset diabetes of the young (MODY)

MODY occurs in approximately 1–2% of people with diabetes but often is not recognised. It is characterised by **early onset**. However, a difference from T1DM is that MODY patients are able to secrete insulin from the β-cells albeit at an insufficient rate or amount to control hyperglycaemia (Chapter 26). MODY is an inherited disorder with **autosomal dominant inheritance caused by a defect of a single gene**. Six gene defects cover 87% of MODY cases in the UK. They are: glucokinase (MODY2) (Chapter 26) and the transcription factors HNF4-α (MODY1), HNF1-α (MODY3), IPF1 (MODY4), HNF1-β (MODY5) and Neuro D1 (MODY6).

(The oxymoron "maturity onset diabetes of the young" was coined in 1974 when "maturity onset diabetes" described what is now T2DM. Logically, using modern nomenclature, MODY should be "T2DMY.)

Glucose Toxicity

Glucose is an important fuel for all tissues and is essential for red blood cells. Ironically, prolonged exposure of cells to **excessive concentrations of glucose can be harmful** through the following mechanisms.

Osmotic Effects

The **hypertonic** effect of high glucose concentrations in the extracellular fluid causes **water** to be drawn **from cells into** the **extracellular fluid**, thence into the **blood** and **excretion** in the **urine,** resulting in **dehydration**.

β-cell damage caused by free radicals

High concentrations of glucose in β-cells result in **enhanced oxidative phosphorylation** which generates increased amounts of reactive oxygen species (**ROS**) causing **oxidative stress** (Chapters 18, 19) and **loss of β-cell function**. The consequence is reduced ability to secrete insulin resulting in hyperglycaemia and thus a **vicious cycle** of **hyperglycaemia/ROS/β-cell dysfunction** ensues **exacerbating** the **diabetes**.

Glycation of proteins

This describes the **non-enzymatic** reaction between **glucose** (and other reducing sugars) with free N-terminal α-amino groups or the ϵ-**amino group of lysyl** residues in proteins which is a normal, but undesirable, ongoing process. **NB Although the reactant is glucose, the product is a fructosamine** (Fig. 33.1). Hyperglycaemia allows glucose to react with proteins in the plasma and tissues, resulting in the accumulation of **glycated products**. Over periods of months and years, these form **advanced glycation end products (AGEs)** which **cross-link** long-lived proteins, e.g. **collagen** resulting in dysfunction and the pathogenesis of **diabetic complications** such as vascular stiffening, hypertension, nephropathy and retinopathy.

(*NB **The nomenclature is confused.** In the 1970s the term **glycosylation** was used for the reaction of **carbohydrates** with protein. Later it was recommended that **glycosylation** be reserved for the reaction of **glucose** with protein while **glycation** means the reaction of **any carbohydrate** with protein.*)

Glycated plasma proteins: fructosamine (also known as glycated serum protein (GSP), glycated albumin)

HbA_{1c} (see below) is a fructosamine however, in clinical practice the term "**fructosamine**" is usually reserved for **glycated serum proteins**. **Albumin**, the principal protein in plasma, and the other plasma proteins are glycated when exposed to hyperglycaemia, producing fructosamine residues. Since the half-life of albumin is 19 days, measurement of fructosamine gives an estimation of **average glycaemic control** over the previous **2–3 weeks**.

Table 33.1 Approximate relationship between $\%HbA_{1c}$ and the average plasma glucose concentration based on population studies and should be used with caution in cases of individual patients.

HbA_{1c} (% of total Hb)	Equivalent average plasma glucose concentration	
	mMol/l	mg/dl
6%	8.1	145
7%	10.0	180
8%	11.9	215
9%	13.9	250
10%	15.8	285
11%	17.8	320
12%	19.7	355

Haemoglobin (HbA_{1c})

HbA_{1c} (the best known glycated protein) is a minor component of haemoglobin, formed during the 17-week lifetime of red blood cells when glucose reacts non-enzymatically with the exposed α-amino group of the N-terminal valine of β-globin, forming a fructosamine residue. **The amount of HbA_{1c} formed is determined by the cumulative exposure to the plasma glucose concentration.** Therefore measurement of HbA_{1c} provides an estimation of the time-averaged glucose concentration during the **8-week period** prior to testing (Table 33.1).

Alcohol metabolism: hypoglycaemia, hyperlactataemia and steatosis

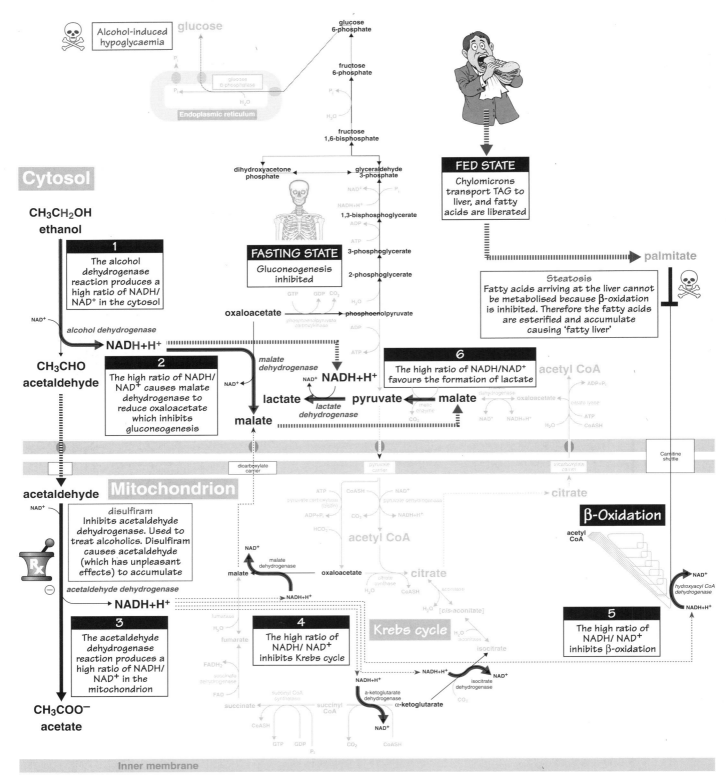

Figure 34.1 Alcohol metabolism.

Ethanol metabolism

Although moderate consumption of ethanol has health benefits, excessive intake causes disease. Ethanol is rapidly metabolised by **alcohol dehydrogenase** in the **cytosol** to form **acetaldehyde**. This requires the coenzyme NAD^+ which is reduced to NADH and results in a **high ratio of NADH/NAD$^+$ in the cytosol**. Subsequently, acetaldehyde is transported into the mitochondrion where it is oxidised by **acetaldehyde dehydrogenase** to **acetate,** which results in a **high mitochondrial ratio of NADH/NAD$^+$**. This elevation of NADH/NAD$^+$ ratios causes the following metabolic consequences of ethanol abuse.

Hypoglycaemia

The high cytosolic ratio of NADH/NAD$^+$ favours reduction of oxaloacetate to malate redirecting this gluconeogenic precursor away from gluconeogenesis. Anyone who has had a social drink after fasting for a few hours will be familiar with the unpleasant consequences of the fall in blood glucose concentration (remember glucose is the preferred fuel for the brain: a fact which will not be forgotten by my friend Keith*). However, for the habitual alcoholic who regularly neglects food and abuses ethanol the hypoglycaemia can be severe and cause coma.

By an extraordinary coincidence, while writing this section my friend Keith phoned to say he had just had an accident caused by alcohol-induced hypoglycaemia! He is a busy plant nurseryman and after a hectic day (minimal breakfast, skipped lunch, much physical exercise, no evening meal; all contriving to exhaust his liver glycogen reserves) he rushed to sing in an evening performance with his choral society. He had a convivial glass of wine before the show. During the programme he began to sweat, felt dizzy and fell, not alas forwards into the warm embrace of the sopranos, but backwards off the podium. He awoke on the way to hospital with a fractured fibula!

Hyperlactataemia

Another consequence of the high ratio of cytosolic NADH/NAD$^+$ described above is that lactate dehydrogenase reduces pyruvate to lactate (Fig. 34.1). Moreover, the malate formed as described above is also metabolised to lactate. Therefore ethanol abuse causes hyperlactataemia.

Inhibition of Krebs cycle

Figure 34.1 shows that the high ratio of NADH/NAD$^+$ in the mitochondrion favours reduction of oxaloacetate to malate in the **malate dehydrogenase** reaction. It also restricts the oxidation in the **α-ketoglutarate dehydrogenase** and **isocitrate dehydrogenase** reactions. The result is that **Krebs cycle is inhibited**.

Steatosis

Steatosis (fatty liver) is a metabolic consequence of ethanol abuse. This results from a high mitochondrial ratio of NADH/NAD$^+$ which prevents β-oxidation of fatty acids.

Figure 34.1 shows that acetaldehyde is metabolised in liver mitochondria by **acetaldehyde dehydrogenase** to form **acetate**; and NAD$^+$ forms NADH resulting in a high ratio of NADH/NAD$^+$. This high ratio of NADH/NAD$^+$ prevents oxidation by the **hydroxyacyl CoA dehydrogenase** reaction, therefore **β-oxidation is inhibited**.

Meanwhile, the liver receives fatty acids from dietary lipids. Since these fatty acids cannot be used for β-oxidation, they are esterified and accumulate in the liver as triacylglycerol (TAG), a condition known as steatosis.

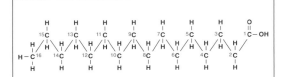

Figure 35.1 Glycerol. A carbohydrate that forms the "backbone" of triacylglycerols (TAGs).

Figure 35.2 Palmitic acid (hexadecanoic acid). A C_{16} saturated fatty acid, i.e. it has 16 carbon atoms, all of which (apart from the C1 carboxylic acid group) are **fully saturated** with hydrogen.

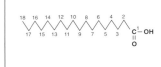

Figure 35.3 Stearic acid (octadecanoic acid). A C_{18} saturated fatty acid, i.e. it has 18 carbon atoms, all of which (apart from the C1 carboxylic acid group) are **fully saturated** with hydrogen. This simplified representation of the structure does not show the hydrogen atoms.

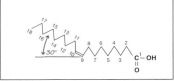

Figure 35.4 *cis*-Oleic acid. A $C_{18:1}$ **mono**-unsaturated fatty acid, i.e. it has **one** double bond at C9, and so the carbon atoms C9 and C10 are not saturated with their full capacity of two hydrogen atoms each. NB The double bond creates a 30° angle. (*cis*- and *trans*- are defined in Fig. 35.14).

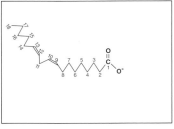

Figure 35.5 Linoleic acid. A $C_{18:2}$ poly-unsaturated fatty acid, i.e. it has 18 carbon atoms and two *cis*-unsaturated bonds at C9 and C12.

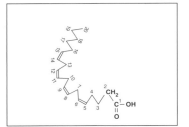

Figure 35.7 Arachidonic acid. A $C_{20:4}$ poly-unsaturated fatty acid i.e. it has 20 carbon atoms and four *cis*-unsaturated bonds at C5, C8, C11 and C14.
NB Arachidonic acid is sometimes mispronounced "arach **nid** onic". Note that it is derived from peanuts (ground nuts) (Greek *arakos*) and NOT from spiders (arachnids)!

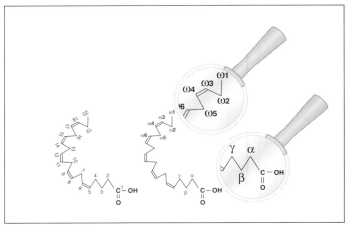

Figure 35.8 Eicosapentaenoic acid (EPA) A $C_{20:5}$ poly-unsaturated fatty acid, i.e. it has 20 carbon atoms and five *cis*-unsaturated bonds at C5, C8, C11, C14 and C17. **Nomenclature**: NB There is an alternative system for identifying the carbon atoms of fatty acids which is popular with nutritionists and uses Greek letters. The carboxylic acid group is ignored and the next carbon is **α**-, then **β**-, **γ**-, etc. until the last carbon which is the last letter of the Greek alphabet, **ω**-. The system then counts backwards from ω, so we have **ω1**, **ω2**, **ω3**, etc. Thus EPA, which is an essential fatty acid found in fish oil, is classified as a **ω3 fatty acid**. *The chemists, (who claim to be the prima donnas of nomenclature) prefer to label the last carbon "n", so chemists refer to n1, n2, n3, etc.).*

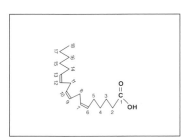

Figure 35.6 γ-Linolenic acid. A $C_{18:3}$ poly-unsaturated fatty acid, i.e. it has 18 carbon atoms and three *cis*-unsaturated bonds at C6, C9 and C12.

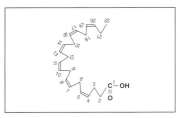

Figure 35.9 Docosahexaenoic acid (DHA). A $C_{22:6}$ poly-unsaturated fatty acid, i.e. it has 22 carbon atoms and six *cis*-unsaturated bonds at C4, C7, C10, C13, C16 and C20.
DHA is an essential fatty acid found in fish oil, and is a **ω3 fatty acid**.

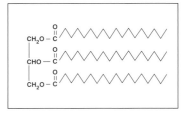

Figure 35.10 Triacylglycerol (TAG or triglyceride). TAG consists of **three** fatty **acyl** groups esterified with a **glycerol** backbone, hence the name **tri acyl glycerol**. The fatty acids can vary but in the example shown all three are **stearic** acid so this TAG is called "**tristearin**". (*In clinical circles the term "**triglyceride**" is commonly used. This incorrectly suggests that the molecule comprises "three glycerols" and so has been rejected by chemists.*)

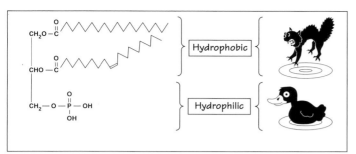

Figure 35.11 Phosphatidic acid. This is the "parent" molecule of the phospholipids. Like triacylglycerol, it has a glycerol backbone but instead comprises two fatty acyl groups and one phosphate group. When this phosphate reacts with OH groups of compounds such as choline, ethanolamine, serine or inositol, phospholipids are formed known as **phosphatidylcholine**, **phosphatidylethanolamine**, **phosphatidylserine** and **phosphatidylinositol**.

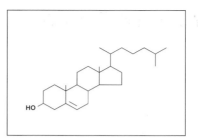

Figure 35.12 Cholesterol.

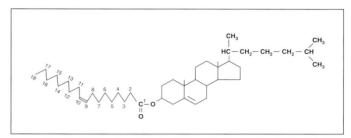

Figure 35.13 Cholesteryl ester. When cholesterol is esterified with a fatty acid, cholesteryl ester is formed.

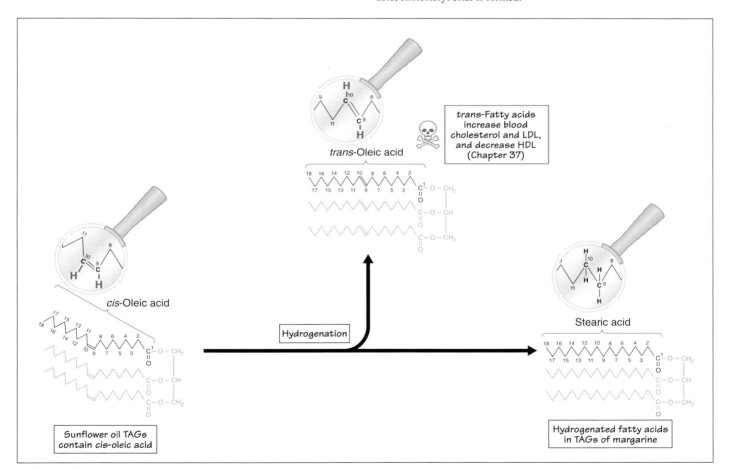

Figure 35.14 *cis*- and *trans*-fatty acids. The terms *cis*- and *trans*-refers to the position of molecules around a double bond. In ***cis***-oleic acid, the hydrogen atoms are on the **same side** of the double bond, whereas in ***trans***-oleic acid, the hydrogen atoms are on **opposite sides** of the double bond. (Think of transatlantic, opposite sides of the Atlantic Ocean.)

Notice that *trans*-fatty acids do not have the 30° angle in their chain. The result is that, although they are unsaturated, they are both structurally and physiologically more like saturated fatty acids. Unfortunately, *trans*-fatty acids can be formed in the hydrogenation process during margarine manufacture which converts the fatty acyl groups of TAG in sunflower oil (a fluid) to (solid) margarine.

36 Phospholipids I: phospholipids and sphingolipids

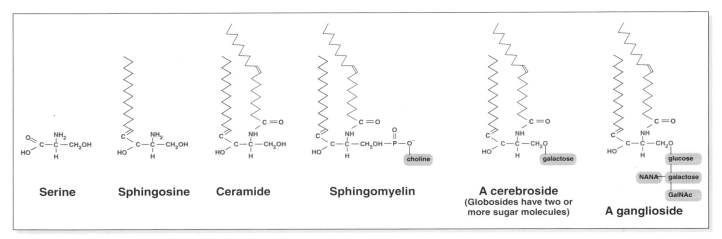

Phosphatidic acid   **Phosphatidylserine**   **Phosphatidyl-ethanolamine**   **Phosphatidylcholine (lecithin)**   **Phosphatidylinositol**

Figure 36.1 Structure of phospholipids.

Serine   **Sphingosine**   **Ceramide**   **Sphingomyelin**   **A cerebroside** (Globosides have two or more sugar molecules)   **A ganglioside**

Figure 36.2 Structure of sphingolipids.

Phospholipids

Phospholipids are important components of cell membranes and lipoproteins (Chapter 37). They are **amphipathic** compounds, i.e. they have an affinity for both aqueous and non-aqueous environments. The **hydrophobic** part of the molecule associates with **hydrophobic, lipid molecules**, while the **hydrophilic** part of the molecule associates with **water**. In this way, phospholipids are compounds that form bridges between water and lipids.

The parent molecule of the phospholipid family is **phosphatidic acid** (Fig. 36.1). It consists of **glycerol** "backbone" to which are esterified **two fatty acyl molecules** (stearic acid is shown here) and phosphoric acid. The later produces a **phosphate** which is free to react with the hydroxyl groups of **serine, ethanolamine, choline** or **inositol** to form **phosphatidylserine, phosphatidylethanolamine, phosphatidylcholine** or **phosphatidylinositol**, respectively.

Phosphatidylcholine

This is also known as **lecithin** and is frequently used in food as an emul-

sifying agent whereby it causes lipids to associate with water molecules.

Respiratory distress syndrome

Respiratory distress syndrome (RDS) is a common problem in premature infants. The immature lung fails to produce **dipalmitoyllecithin** which is a surfactant. RDS occurs when the alveoli collapse inwards after expiration and adhere under the prevailing surface tension (atelectasis). The function of dipalmitoyllecithin is to reduce the surface tension and permit expansion of the alveoli on inflation. Assessment of the maturity of foetal lung function can be made by measuring the ratio of **lecithin** to **sphingomyelin** (the **L/S ratio**) in amniotic fluid.

Phosphatidylinositol

This is the parent molecule of the phosphoinositides, e.g. **phosphatidylinositol 3,4,5-tris phosphate (PIP$_3$)** which is involved in insulin-stimulated intracellular signal transduction (Chapter 29).

82 Phospholipids I: phospholipids and sphingolipids

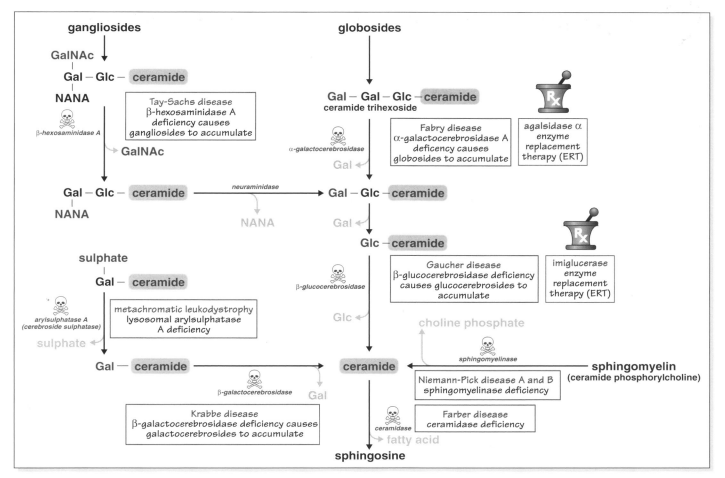

Figure 36.3 Degradation of sphingolipids and the sphingolipidoses.

Sphingolipids

Sphingolipids are major components of cell membranes and are especially abundant in myelin. They are similar to the glycerol-containing phospholipids described above except their hydrophilic "backbone" is **serine** (Fig. 36.2 *opposite*). They are derived from **sphingosine** which is formed when palmitoyl CoA loses a carbon atom as CO_2 in a reaction with serine. Sphingosine is *N*-acylated to form **ceramide**, which is the group common to the sphingolipids, e.g. **sphingomyelin** and the carbohydrate-containing **cerebrosides** and **gangliosides**. The **sphingolipidoses** are a group of lysosomal disorders characterised by impaired breakdown of the sphingolipids (Fig. 36.3). The lipid products that accumulate cause the disease.

Sphingomyelin

The addition of phosphorylcholine to ceramide produces **sphingomyelin** (Fig. 36.2). Sphingomyelin (also known as ceramide phosphorylcholine) is analogous to phosphatidylcholine.

Cerebrosides

When ceramide combines with a monosaccharide such as **galactose (Gal)**, or **glucose (Glc)** the product is a **cerebroside**, e.g. **galactocerebroside** (or galactosylceramide) (Fig. 36.2) or **glucocerebroside** (or glucosylceramide). Cerebrosides are also known as "**mono**glycosylceramides". **Globosides** are cerebrosides containing two or more sugars.

Gaucher disease

Gaucher disease, the most prevalent lysosomal storage disease, is an autosomal recessive disorder caused by lysosomal deficiency of **β-glucocerebrosidase (GBA)** (Fig. 36.3). This results in excessive accumulation of glucocerebroside in the brain, liver, bone marrow and spleen. Type 1 Gaucher disease (non-neuronopathic form) can be treated by **enzyme replacement therapy (ERT)** with recombinant β-glucocerebrosidase. In the future, Gaucher disease is a potential candidate for gene therapy by inserting the GBA gene into haemopoetic stem cells.

Gangliosides and globosides

When ceramide combines with **oligosaccharides** and **N-acetyl-neuraminic** acid (**NANA** also known as **sialic acid**) the **gangliosides** are formed. Gangliosides comprise approximately 5% of brain lipids.

Fabry disease

Fabry disease is a rare X-linked lysosomal disorder caused by deficience of **α-galactocerebrosidase A** (Fig. 36.3). This results in the accumulation of globoside **ceramide trihexoside, (CTH)** (also known as **globotriaosylceramide**) throughout the body causing progressive renal, cardiovascular and cerebrovascular disease. Since 2002 enzyme replacement therapy using recombinant α-galactocerebrosidase has been available.

Phospholipids II: micelles, liposomes, lipoproteins and membranes

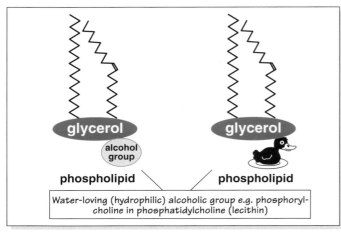

Figure 37.1 Phospholipids. A cartoon representation of a phospholipid is shown in which the **hydrophilic** (**water-loving**) part of the molecule (e.g. phosphorylserine or phosphorylcholine) is represented by a water-loving duck.

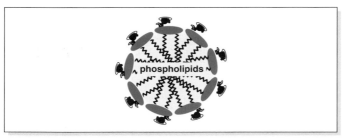

Figure 37.2 Micelles. When phospholipids are mixed with water, they associate to form a micelle. This is a spherical structure where the **hydrophobic** parts of the molecule associate in an inner core while the **hydrophilic** parts of the molecule associate with the surrounding water.

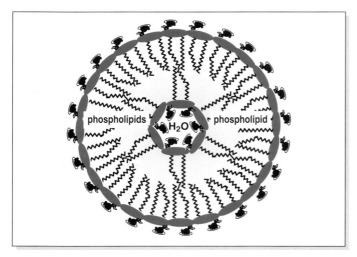

Figure 37.3 Liposomes. Liposomes are small artificial vesicles which are formed when phospholipids and water are subjected to high-shear mixing or to vigorous agitation by an ultrasonic probe. Liposomes can be used to encapsulate hydrophilic drugs and are used for delivery of some anticancer drugs. They are also used to deliver cosmetics.

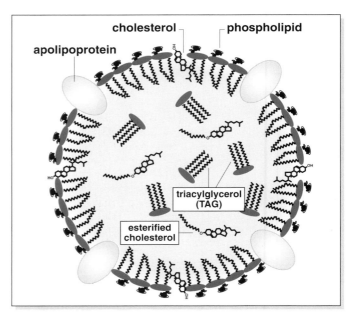

Figure 37.4 Lipoproteins. Lipoproteins are macromolecular complexes used by the body to transport lipids in the blood. They are characterised by an outer coat of phospholipids and proteins which encloses an inner core of hydrophobic TAG and cholesteryl ester. Lipoproteins are classified according to the way they behave on centrifugation. This in turn corresponds to their relative densities which depends on the proportion of (high density) protein to (low density) lipid in their structure. For example, **high density lipoproteins (HDLs)** consist of **50% protein** and have the highest density while **chylomicrons (1% protein)** and **very low density proteins (VLDLs)** have the lowest density.

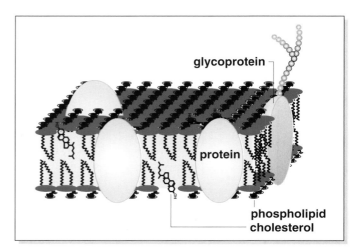

Figure 37.5 Membranes. The membranes in mammalian cells are composed of a mixture of phospholipids, proteins and cholesterol, which organises to form a bimolecular sheet.

Table 37.1 Apolipoproteins and their properties. The apolipoproteins are located in the outer protein-containing layer of lipoproteins. They confer on the lipoproteins their identifying characteristics.

ApoA1	**In HDL (90% total protein), chylomicrons (3% total protein)**
	High affinity for cholesterol, removes cholesterol from cells
	Activates LCAT
ApoB48	**In chylomicrons**
	Made in intestine when TAG biosynthesis is active during fat absorption.
ApoB100	**In VLDL (and in IDL and LDL, which are derived from VLDL)**
	Made in hepatocytes when TAG and cholesterol biosynthesis is active
	Binds to receptor
ApoC2	**In chylomicrons and VLDL**
	Activates lipoprotein lipase when the chylomicrons and VLDL arrive at their target tissue
ApoE	**In chylomicrons, VLDL and HDL**
	Binds to receptor

Table 37.2 Plasma lipoproteins. As shown in Fig. 37.4 lipoproteins are spherical structures with a **hydrophilic exterior** and a **hydrophobic** (lipid-containing) **core**. Their function is to transport lipids in the hydrophilic environment of the blood. The outer surface of lipoproteins is rich in phospholipids and apolipoproteins (Table 37.1) which confer upon the lipoproteins many of their specific properties.

	Chylomicron	Very low density lipoprotein (VLDL)	Intermediate density lipoprotein (IDL)	Low density lipoprotein (LDL)	High density lipoprotein (HDL)
Plasma lipoproteins					
Origin	Intestine	Liver	Derived from VLDLs	Derived from VLDLs and IDLs	Intestine and liver
Function	Transport dietary TAG and cholesterol from the intestines to the periphery	Forward transport of endogenous TAG and cholesterol from liver to periphery	Precursor of LDLs	Cholesterol transport	1 Reverse transport of cholesterol from periphery to the liver. 2 Stores apoprotein C2 and apoprotein E which it supplies to chylomicrons and VLDLs 3 Scavenges apolipoproteins released from chylomicrons and VLDL following lipoprotein lipase activity in the capillaries
Components of lipoproteins (%)					
TAG	90	65	30	10	2
Cholesterol/ester	5	13	40	45	18
Phospholipids	4	12	20	25	30
Proteins	1	10	10	20	50

38 Metabolism of carbohydrate and fat to cholesterol

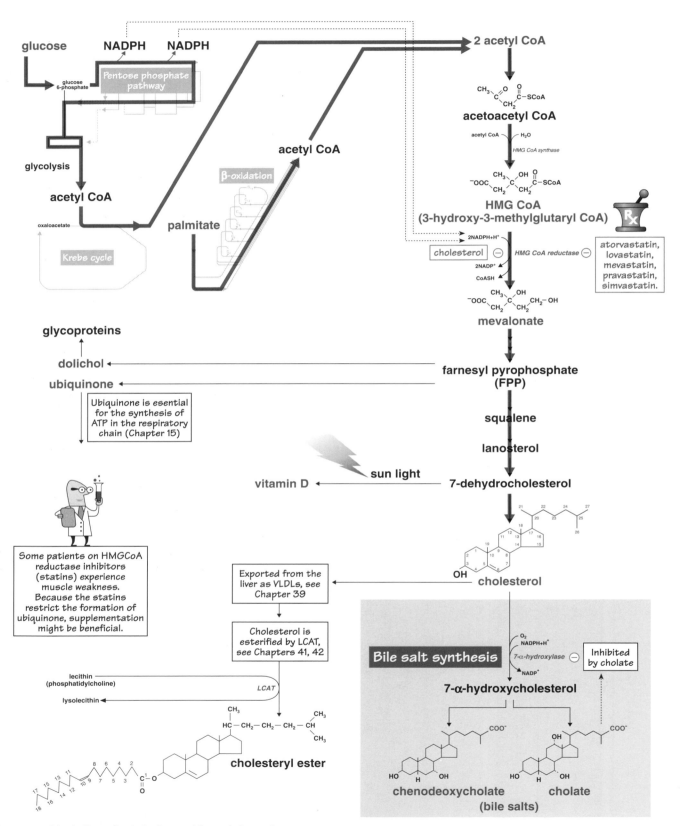

Figure 38.1 Metabolism of carbohydrate and fat to cholesterol.

Cholesterol: friend or foe?

Cholesterol is a lipid named from the Greek roots *chole* (bile), *ster* (solid) and **ol** (because it has an alcohol group). It is normally found in bile but if present at supersaturated concentrations, it crystallises out to form "solid bile", i.e. gall stones. Cholesterol has many important functions, for example it is a **component of cell membranes**, and is a precursor of the **bile salts** (Fig. 38.1) and the steroid hormones (**aldosterone, cortisol, testosterone, progesterone** and **oestrogens** (Chapter 43)). However, if present in excessive amounts in the blood, cholesterol is deposited in arterial walls causing atherosclerosis. Cholesterol can also be deposited as yellow deposits in soft tissues causing tendon xanthomata (Greek *xantho-*, yellow), palmar xanthomata, xanthelasmata and corneal arcus.

Biosynthesis of cholesterol

Cholesterol can be made *de novo* from dietary carbohydrate or TAG

Cholesterol is made in the liver from glucose via the pentose phosphate pathway (which generates NADPH) and glycolysis which produces acetyl CoA, (Fig. 38.1). Fatty acids can also be oxidised by β-oxidation to acetyl CoA. Acetyl CoA is then metabolised to 3-hydroxy-3-methylglutaryl CoA (HMGCoA) which is reduced by NADPH in the presence of **HMGCoA reductase** (the regulatory enzyme for cholesterol synthesis) to form **mevalonate**. Mevalonate is then metabolised via more than two dozen intermediates (not shown) to form cholesterol.

HMGCoA reductase regulates cholesterol biosynthesis

Clearly, cholesterol biosynthesis must be regulated to prevent the diseases associated with **hypercholesterolaemia** and the regulation of HMGCoA reductase has been the subject of much research. Three mechanisms are used: (i) HMGCoA reductase is down-regulated by cholesterol (**feedback inhibition**), (ii) insulin stimulates HMGCoA reductase while glucagon inhibits it (both hormonal effects are mediated by **protein phosphorylation cascades** similar to those used to regulate glycogen metabolism (Chapters 10, 29)) and (iii) cholesterol **restricts transcription** thereby decreasing the formation of mRNA needed for synthesis of HMGCoA reductase (Chapter 10).

Pharmacological treatment of hypercholesterolaemia using statins

The **statins** are reversible inhibitors of HMGCoA reductase and inhibit cholesterol biosynthesis. The resulting fall in cellular cholesterol concentration increases expression of LDL receptors, therefore more LDL cholesterol is removed from the blood. By lowering blood concentrations of LDL cholesterol statins they have made a dramatic impact on the prevention of cardiovascular disease. NB The statins restrict the formation of **mevalonate** and consequently the formation of all other downstream intermediates involved in cholesterol biosynthesis might also be restricted. In particular, the production of **farnesyl pyrophosphate** and its product **ubiquinone** will be decreased. Since ubiquinone is an essential component of the respiratory chain (Chapters 15–17), which is needed for ATP biosynthesis, it is possible that the statins could compromise the ATP production needed for energy metabolism in exercising muscle. This could be responsible for the muscle cramps or weakness experienced by some patients treated with statins and it has been suggested these patients might benefit from supplementation with ubiquinone (also known as coenzyme Q_{10}).

Ubiquinone, dolichol and vitamin D are important by-products of the cholesterol biosynthetic pathway

It has been mentioned above that **ubiquinone** is an important by-product of cholesterol biosynthesis. However, note that other by-products are **dolichol** (needed for glycoprotein biosynthesis) and **vitamin D** (Chapter 53).

Forward transport of cholesterol from the liver to peripheral tissues

Once cholesterol has been made in the liver, it must be transported to the periphery where it is needed. However, since it is not soluble in the aqueous environment of the blood it must be packaged in very low density lipoproteins (**VLDLs**) for transport to the tissues (Chapter 39). *(NB Dietary cholesterol is similarly transported from the gut to the periphery in hydrophilic spheres known as **chylomicrons** (Chapter 37)).*

Reverse transport of cholesterol from peripheral tissues to the liver

Cholesterol is removed from peripheral tissues by high density lipoproteins (HDLs) (Chapter 39) which are frequently praised as being "good lipoproteins".

Biosynthesis of bile salts

The bile salts (**chenodeoxycholate** and **cholate**) are needed to emulsify lipids prior to intestinal absorption. Their biosynthesis from cholesterol is regulated by **7 α-hydroxylase**.

VLDL and LDL metabolism ("forward" cholesterol transport)

Transport to and from the liver

The liver is organised into collections of cells known as lobules (Fig. 39.1). Each lobule receives blood from two sources. Like other organs, it receives oxygenated blood (via the hepatic artery). However, it also receives the venous blood which drains from the gut. The liver is unique in having an afferent venous supply, namely via the hepatic portal vein. This vein transports many products of digestion such as glucose from the gut to the liver. (**NB Chylomicrons are not transported via the portal vein.** They proceed via the lymphatic system before entering the thoracic duct and joining the blood stream.) The products of liver metabolism leave by two routes. Most products leave by the hepatic vein, which is in the centre of a liver lobule. However, certain products such as the bile salts are excreted via the bile ducts.

Cholesterol synthesis and transport

Cholesterol is synthesised from glucose by the liver (Chapter 38). Some of the cholesterol is esterified with fatty acids in a reaction catalysed by **a**cyl CoA–cholesterol–**a**cyl **t**ransferase (**ACAT**) to form **cholesteryl ester** (Fig. 39.2). This is hydrophobic and with its hydrophobic associate, the triacylglycerols, is stored in the core of the **nascent VLDL** particles. The nascent VLDLs leave the liver via the hepatic vein and progress to the

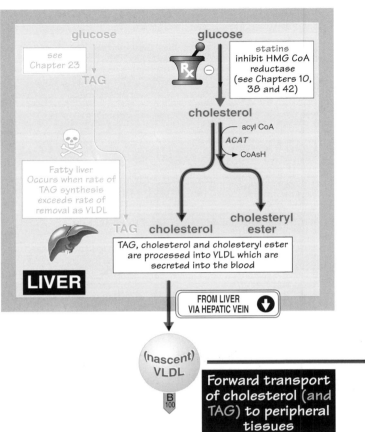

Figure 39.2 "Forward transport" of cholesterol to the peripheral tissues and its excretion as bile salts.

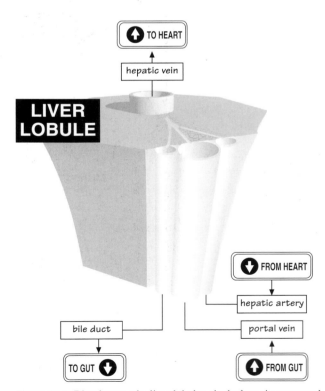

Figure 39.1 Blood enters the liver lobules via the hepatic artery and the portal vein. It leaves via the hepatic vein.

periphery. In the peripheral capillaries, lipoprotein lipase removes much of the triacylglycerol content by hydrolysing them to fatty acids and glycerol leaving the remnant of the VLDL, known as an **intermediate density lipoprotein (IDL)**, relatively rich in cholesterol. Removal of apoE produces LDL particles which are cleared by binding to the LDL receptor. Here they are degraded to their constituent components. The cholesterol produced can be cleared from the body by conversion to bile salts (Chapter 38) which are excreted from the liver via the bile duct into the intestine. A substantial proportion of the bile salts is reabsorbed and recirculated via the liver in the "**enterohepatic circulation**".

Disorder of LDL metabolism
Type 2 hyperlipidaemia

Patients with **familial hypercholesterolaemia** have very high serum cholesterol concentrations. They die at a young age from ischaemic heart disease if they are not treated. The disorder is due to failure to produce functional **LDL receptors**. The deficit of LDL receptors results in a failure to clear LDL from the blood. The LDLs accumulate and cause atherosclerosis.

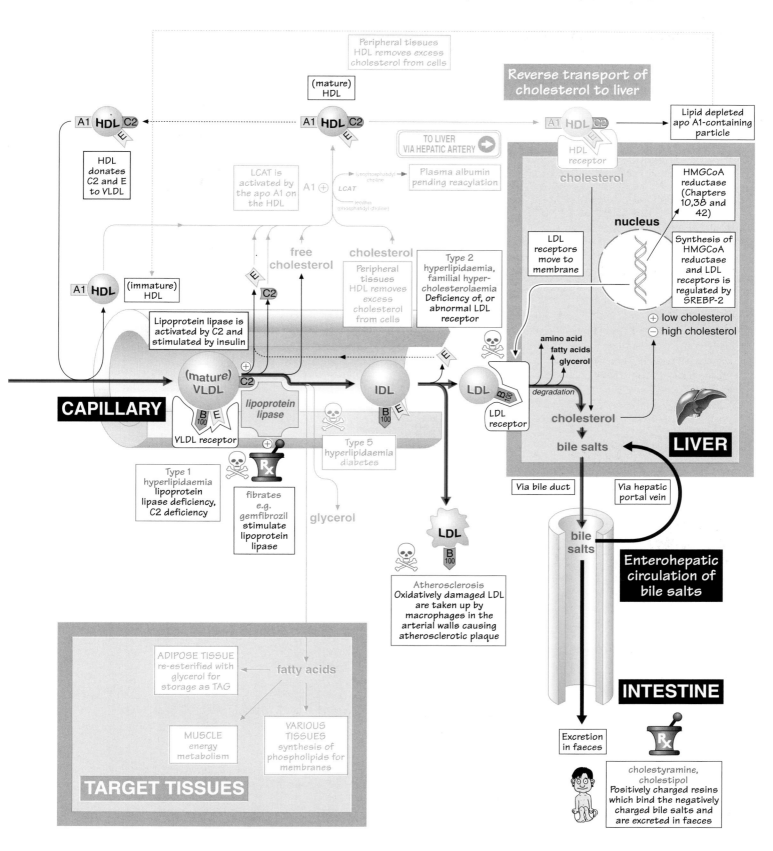

40 VLDL and LDL metabolism (endogenous triacylglycerol transport)

Biosynthesis of triacylglycerols (TAGs) in liver

We have seen in Chapter 23 how glucose can be metabolised to fatty acids. The fatty acids are then esterified to form TAGs. The newly formed TAGs must not be allowed to accumulate in the liver (otherwise a fatty liver results as when geese are force-fed to make *pâté de foie gras*). The hydrophobic globules of fat must be transported in the aqueous environment of the blood. This is done by enveloping them with a hydrophilic coat of phospholipids and protein to form nascent **v**ery **l**ow **d**ensity **l**ipoproteins (**VLDLs**). The VLDLs leave the liver via the hepatic vein and are transported to the periphery.

Disposal of TAGs in target tissues

The **nascent VLDLs** while *en route* to the target tissues become **mature VLDLs** after receiving from **h**igh **d**ensity **l**ipoproteins (**HDLs**) the apolipoproteins **apoC2** and **apoE**. In the capillaries of the target tissues, the apolipoproteins apoB100 and apoE bind to the VLDL receptor and C2 activates **lipoprotein lipase** (**LPL**), which is further stimulated by insulin. LPL hydrolyses the TAG contained in the VLDLs producing fatty acids and glycerol. Their fate depends on the target tissue: (i) **in adipose tissue** the fatty acids are re-esterified with glycerol reforming TAG for storage; (ii) **in muscle** the fatty acids could be used for energy metabolism; or alternatively (iii) **in various tissues** the fatty acids and glycerol are synthesised to phospholipids for incorporation into cell membranes.

Disposal of intermediate density lipoproteins (IDLs) and low density lipoproteins (LDLs)

Lipoprotein lipase in the capillaries of peripheral tissues acts on VLDLs to form **IDLs** which are metabolised to **LDLs**. In liver ApoB100 of LDL binds to the LDL receptors. These are internalised, and the LDLs are degraded to fatty acids, glycerol, amino acids and cholesterol within the cell.

Disorders of VLDL metabolism

Type 3 hyperlipidaemia (remnant removal disease)

Patients have yellow streaks in the palmar creases of their hand which is pathognomic of type 3 hyperlipidaemia. This is a rare, autosomal recessive condition caused by the production of **abnormal apoE molecules**. Since functional apoE is needed to bind the

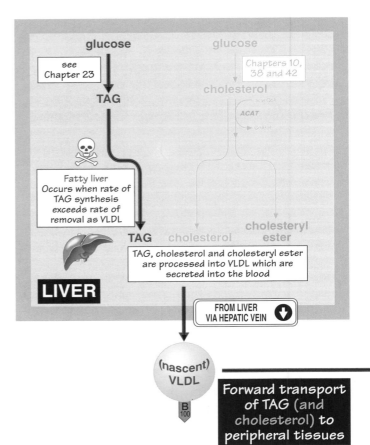

Figure 40.1 VLDL and LDL metabolism.

remnants of VLDL and chylomicrons to the receptor for catabolism, the remnant particles IDLs accumulate. Laboratory tests reveal a "**broad β-band**" on electrophoresis.

Type 4 hyperlipidaemia

This is an autosomal dominant dyslipidaemia characterised by overproduction of TAGs and consequently VLDLs. Serum cholesterol concentrations are normal or slightly raised.

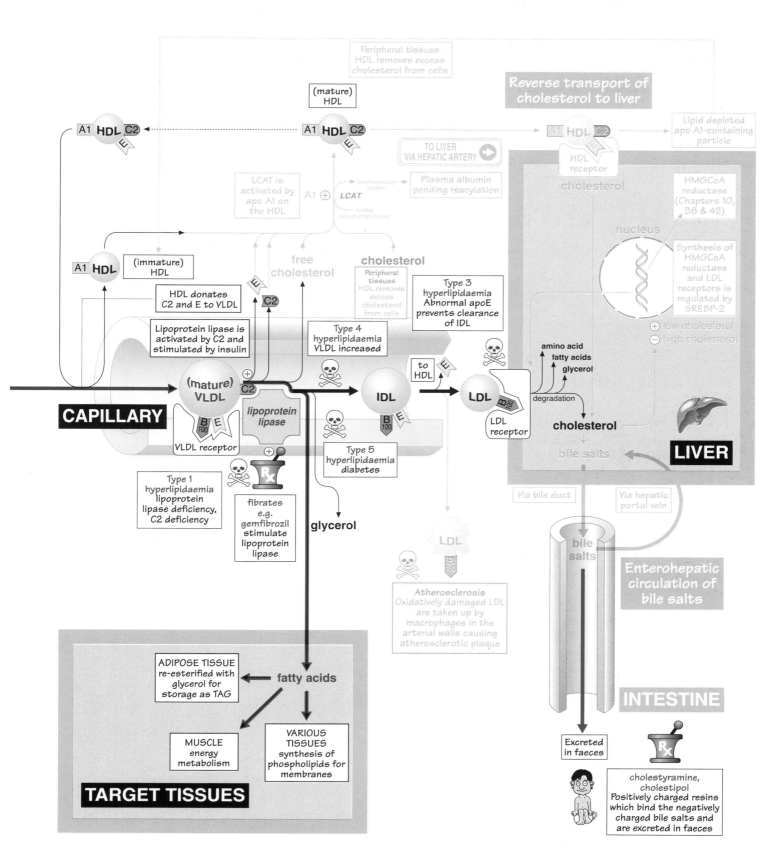

VLDL and LDL metabolism (endogenous triacylglycerol transport) 91

41 HDL metabolism ("reverse" cholesterol transport)

HDL are the "good" lipoproteins that dispose of excess cholesterol

The cholesterol-rich LDL particles are notorious as the "bad guys" of lipoprotein metabolism. On the other hand, HDL particles enjoy the reputation as the "good guys". This is because the function of HDL is to remove surplus cholesterol and transport it to the liver for disposal as bile salts.

HDL scavenges cholesterol from two sources:

1. Lipoprotein lipase activity primarily hydrolyses the triacylglycerol content of lipoproteins to form fatty acids and glycerol. However, in the process it liberates some cholesterol which is incorporated into HDL particles and is transported to the liver for disposal.

2. ABC transporter proteins are a ubiquitous family of proteins characterised by an ATP-**b**inding-**c**assette (**ABC**) motif (Chapter 42). These ATP-binding proteins belong to one of the largest families known to medical science. The bound ATP is hydrolysed in a process coupled to transport of their substrate. One such protein is the cholesterol transporter known as **ABC-A1** (not shown in Fig. 41.1). It is found in many tissues where its function is to transfer excess cholesterol to HDL particles. The HDL particles proceed to the liver for disposal.

Disposal of cholesterol as bile salts

Cholesterol is metabolised to form **bile salts** (Chapter 38) which are excreted in the bile duct. The bile salts emulsify fats in the intestine, which renders them available for hydrolysis by pancreatic lipase which is secreted into the gut. About 95% of the bile salts are absorbed in to the hepatic portal vein and are recycled to the liver by the "**enterohepatic circulation**". About 5% of the bile salts are lost in the faeces.

The enterohepatic circulation can be interrupted by anti-cholesterol agents. These are positively charged resins that bind to the negatively charged bile salts. The resin/bile salt complex is egested in the faeces.

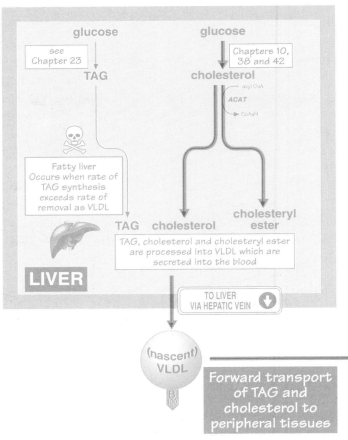

Figure 41.1 HDL metabolism ("reverse" cholesterol transport).

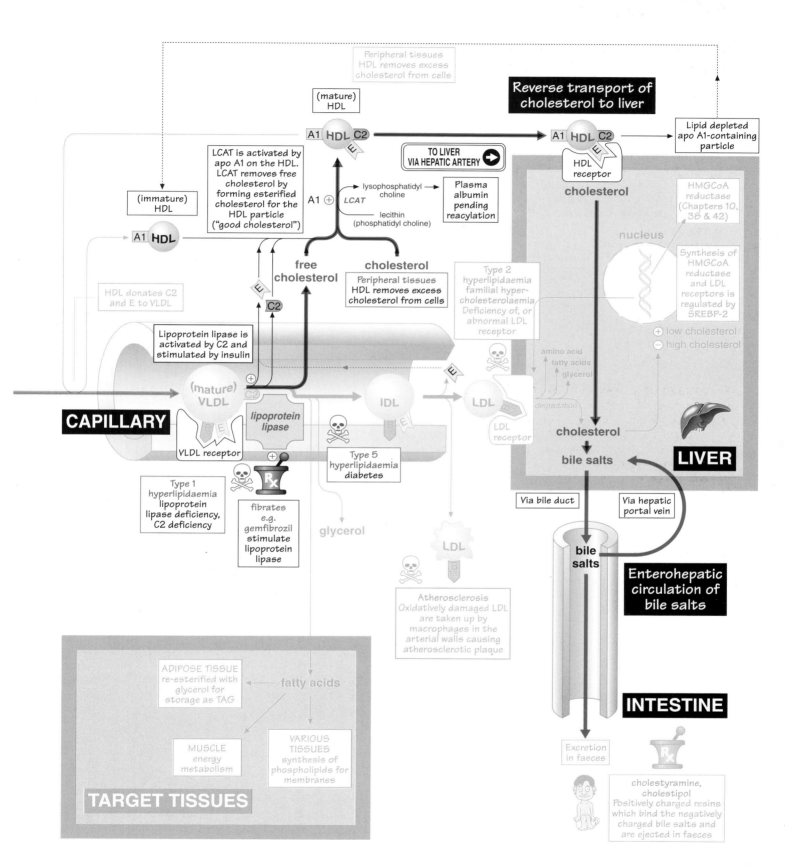

Absorption and disposal of dietary triacylglycerols and cholesterol by chylomicrons

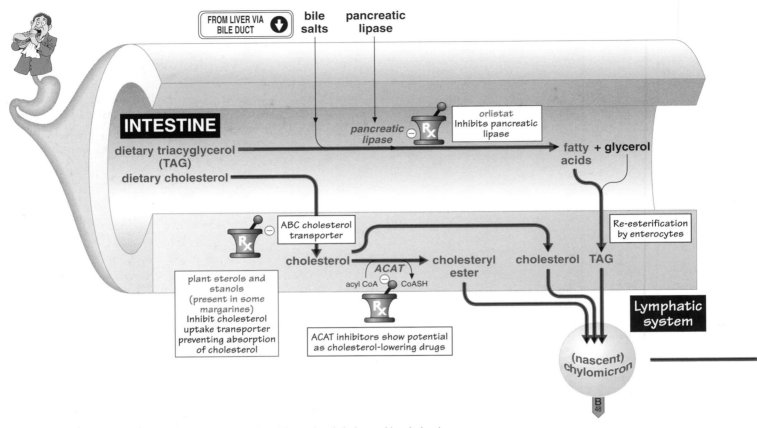

Figure 42.1 Absorption and disposal of dietary triacylglycerol and cholesterol by chylomicrons.

Absorption of dietary triacylglycerols

Dietary triacylglycerols pass through the stomach to the gut where they are emulsified in the presence of the bile salts. Pancreatic lipase is secreted into the gut where it hydrolyses triacylglycerols to fatty acids and glycerol. The fatty acids and glycerol are absorbed by the intestinal cells and re-esterified to triacylglycerols.

Intestinal absorption of cholesterol

Dietary cholesterol is absorbed by **intestinal ABC cholesterol transporter**, (Chapter 41). Once inside the cell, cholesterol is esterified by a**c**yl CoA-**c**holesterol-**a**cyl **t**ransferase (**ACAT**) to form the **hydrophobic** cholesteryl ester. This reaction facilitates and maximises absorption of cholesterol, which is probably an advantage to people deprived of cholesterol-rich food such as meat. Unfortunately, efficient absorption of cholesterol is not an advantage to the affluent. However, margarines enriched with plant sterols have been used to inhibit cholesterol absorption in an attempt to lower blood cholesterol. Research is underway to develop **ACAT inhibitors** which potentially are cholesterol-lowering drugs. Ezetimibe is a new drug which inhibits cholesterol absorption by a mechanism which is not understood.

Chylomicrons

Triacylglycerols and cholesteryl ester are enveloped by a coat of phospholipids and **apoB48** to form **nascent chylomicrons**. These are secreted by the enterocytes into the lymphatic system, which converge to form the thoracic duct. The thoracic duct joins the blood stream in the thorax at the left and right subclavian veins.

Disposal of triacylglycerols

Chylomicrons travel in the blood to the capillaries where they acquire **apoE** and **apoC2** from HDL. On arrival at the target tissues, they bind to lipoprotein lipase and associated, negatively-charged proteoglycans. Lipoprotein lipase is activated by apoC2 and hydrolyses the triacylglycerols to form fatty acids and glycerol. The fate of the fatty acids depends on the type of tissue. In adipose tissue, the fatty acids are re-esterified with the glycerol to reform triacylglycerols which are stored until needed. In muscle, the fatty acids could be used as metabolic fuel.

Disposal of cholesterol

The disruption to the chylomicrons caused by lipoprotein lipase allows cholesterol to be released. This is scavenged by **HDL** which transports the cholesterol for metabolism to bile salts in the liver.

Further reading: Frayn KN (2003) "*Metabolic Regulation: a human perspective*", 2nd ed. Blackwell Publishing, Oxford.

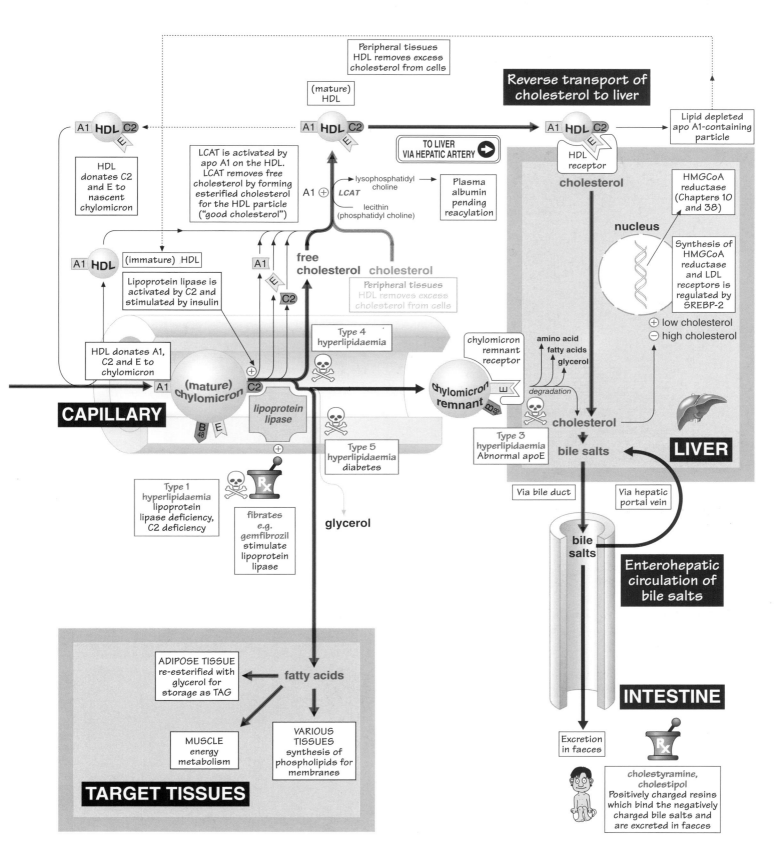

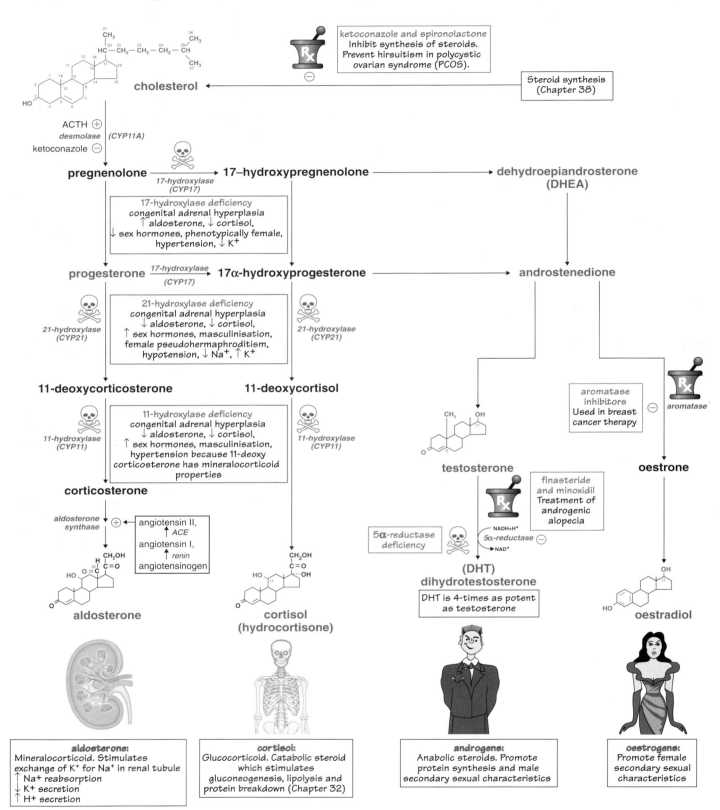

Figure 43.1 Biosynthesis of the steroid hormones.

The steroid hormones

There are four main types of steroid hormone: (i) **mineralocorticoids**, (ii) **glucocorticoids**, (iii) the male sex hormones (**androgens**), and (iv) the female sex hormones (**oestrogens**), (Fig. 43.1). NB **Androstenedione** is the precursor of **both** the androgens and oestrogens. Indeed, a wit once noted that the only difference between Romeo and Juliet was the ketone group on the 3-carbon atom and the methyl group on carbon 10 of the steroid nucleus.

Hyperaldosteronism

Conn's disease is **primary hyperaldosteronism** caused by a rare aldosterone-secreting tumour. Consequently, excessive amounts of potassium and hydrogen ions are lost in the urine resulting in hypocalcaemia and metabolic alkalosis. **Secondary hyperaldosteronism** due to kidney or liver disease is more common.

Adrenocortical insufficiency (Addison's disease)

Addison's disease is a rare, potentially fatal condition due to **insufficient** production of **both aldosterone and cortisol** caused by atrophy of the adrenal glands. It is characterised by low blood pressure, loss of sodium, weight loss and pigmentation of mucosal membranes. Adrenocortical insufficiency also results from pituitary failure with loss of ACTH production.

Hypercortisolism: Cushing's syndrome

Cortisol is secreted by the adrenal **cortex** in response to stress and starvation. It stimulates fat breakdown and also **glucose production** by gluconeogenesis from amino acids derived from tissue proteins. Hence cortisol is a **catabolic steroid** and is secreted during starvation. Natural steroids or synthetic analogues (e.g. dexamethasone) are known as "**glucocorticosteroids**". Secretion of cortisol is regulated by the hypothalamic/pituitary/adrenal axis which respectively secrete **corticotrophin-releasing hormone (CRH)** from the hypothalamus, which stimulates secretion of **adrenocorticotrophic hormone (ACTH)** from the posterior pituitary, which stimulates secretion of **cortisol** from the adrenal cortex. Excessive amounts of cortisol cause Cushing's syndrome, which has four causes: (1) **iatrogenic**, (2) **pituitary adenoma**, (3) **adrenal adenoma/carcinoma**, or (4) **ectopic** production of **ACTH**.

1. Iatrogenic Cushing's syndrome is the most common presentation.
2. The syndrome was first described by Cushing in a patient with a rare primary pituitary adenoma that secreted ACTH. This condition is known as Cushing's disease.
3. Subsequently, patients were described with primary adrenal adenoma (benign)/carcinoma (malignant) in which blood cortisol was increased but ACTH was decreased.
4. Ectopic production of ACTH, for example by small cell lung carcinoma.

Patients with Cushing's syndrome characteristically have a moon-shaped face, thin legs and arms, and truncal obesity due to accumulation of visceral fat (like a pear on match sticks). At first, **accumulation of fat** in the presence of cortisol (a **catabolic** steroid) appears to be counterintuitive. However, hypercortisolism-driven gluconeogenesis increases the blood glucose concentration which increases secretion of insulin. In Cushing's syndrome, cortisol overwhelms insulin rendering it inefficient at reducing the blood glucose concentration. On the other hand, **insulin activity prevails in visceral adipose tissue** where it stimulates expression of **lipoprotein lipase**. This favours lipid accumulation in **visceral** rather than subcutaneous adipose tissue because of the higher blood flow and greater number of adipocytes in the former.

Sex hormones

Impaired androgen synthesis: 5 α-reductase deficiency (5-ARD)

In this condition there is an impaired ability to produce **dihydrotestosterone (DHT)** causing an increased serum ratio of testosterone/DHT (Fig. 43.1). Because DHT is four times as potent as testosterone, genetic males with 5-ARD usually present as neonates with ambiguous genitalia and gender assignment is a major issue.

5α-reductase inhibitors

Finasteride and **minoxidil** are used to treat androgenic alopecia. Finasteride shrinks the prostate in benign prostatic hypertrophy (BPH). **Flutamide** is a testosterone receptor blocker used in prostate carcinoma

Aromatase inhibitors: new drugs for breast cancer

Aromatase inhibitors, e.g. **anastrozole**, **letrozole** and **exemestane**, restrict the formation of oestrogens from androstenedione and are new drugs used to treat breast cancer (Fig. 43.1). In fact, clinical trials of letrozole were so effective that the trials were stopped as it was considered unethical to continue with volunteers on placebo.

44 Urea cycle and overview of amino acid catabolism

Catabolism of amino acids produces ammonium ions (NH₄⁺)

Proteins are hydrolysed in the stomach by pepsin to form amino acids. Further hydrolysis occurs in the intestine. The amino acids are absorbed. Any amino acids in excess of those needed to replace the wear and tear of tissues, and for biosynthesis to hormones, pyrimidines, purines etc, are used for gluconeogenesis, or for energy metabolism. However, catabolism of amino acids generates **ammonium ions (NH₄⁺)**, which are very toxic. Accordingly, NH_4^+ is disposed of by conversion to **urea** which is non-toxic and which is readily excreted via the kidney.

Ammonium ions are metabolised to urea in the urea cycle

Figure 44.1 shows that catabolism of amino acids generates either NH_4^+ directly or **glutamate** which is subsequently deaminated to form NH_4^+. Ammonium ion reacts with **bicarbonate ion** and 2 molecules of **ATP** in a reaction catalysed by **carbamoyl phosphate synthetase (CPS)** to form **carbamoyl phosphate**. This now reacts with **ornithine** to form **citrulline** in the presence of **ornithine transcarbamoylase (OTC)**. **Aspartate** (the vehicle for the second amino group) reacts with **citrulline** to form **argininosuccinate** which is cleaved to produce fumarate and **arginine**. Finally, the arginine is hydrolysed to form **urea** and in the process generates ornithine which is now available to repeat the cycle.

*NB do not confuse the **CPS** mentioned here with **CPS II** which is involved in the synthesis of pyrimidines (Chapter 50).*

Disorders of the urea cycle: OTC deficiency

There are several rare disorders of the urea cycle. However, the most common is **OTC deficiency**, which is an X-linked disease. In severe neonatal forms of the disease, patients rapidly die from ammonium toxicity. However, the disease is variable and some boys have mild forms of the disease. In heterozygous females, the condition varies from being undetectable to a severity that matches that of the boys.

In the 1990s, there was once considerable optimism that OTC deficiency would be an ideal candidate for liver-directed **gene therapy**. Unfortunately, a study of 17 subjects with mild forms of OTC deficiency using an **adenoviral vector** demonstrated little gene transfer and when subject 18 died following complications, the trial was abandoned.

In patients with OTC deficiency, **carbamoyl phosphate** in the presence of **aspartate transcarbamoylase** is diverted to form **orotic acid** (see pyrimidine biosynthesis, Chapter 50) which can be detected in the urine and used to assist with the diagnosis.

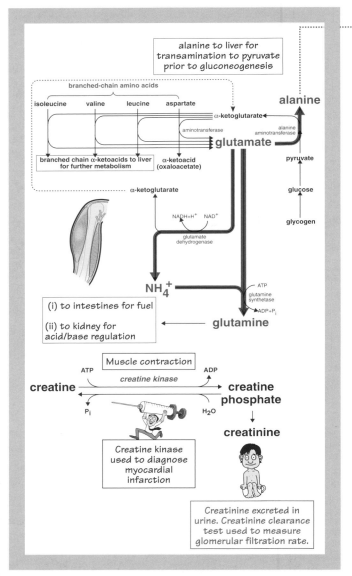

Figure 44.1 An overview of amino acid catabolism and the detoxification of NH_4^+ by forming urea.

Creatine

Arginine is the precursor of **creatine**, which combines with ATP to form **creatine phosphate** (Chapter 14). Creatine is excreted as **creatinine**.

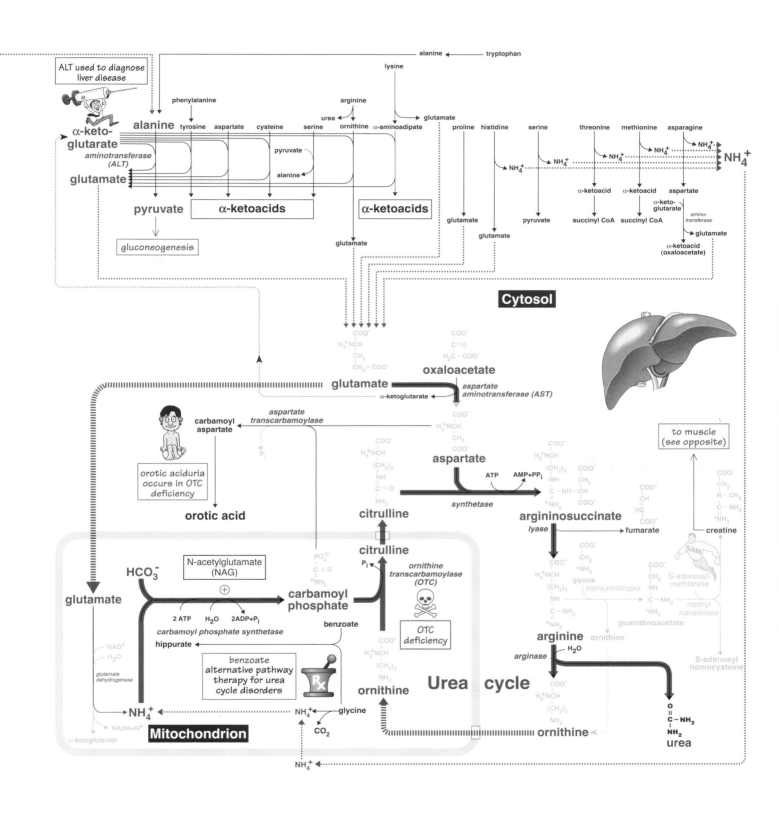

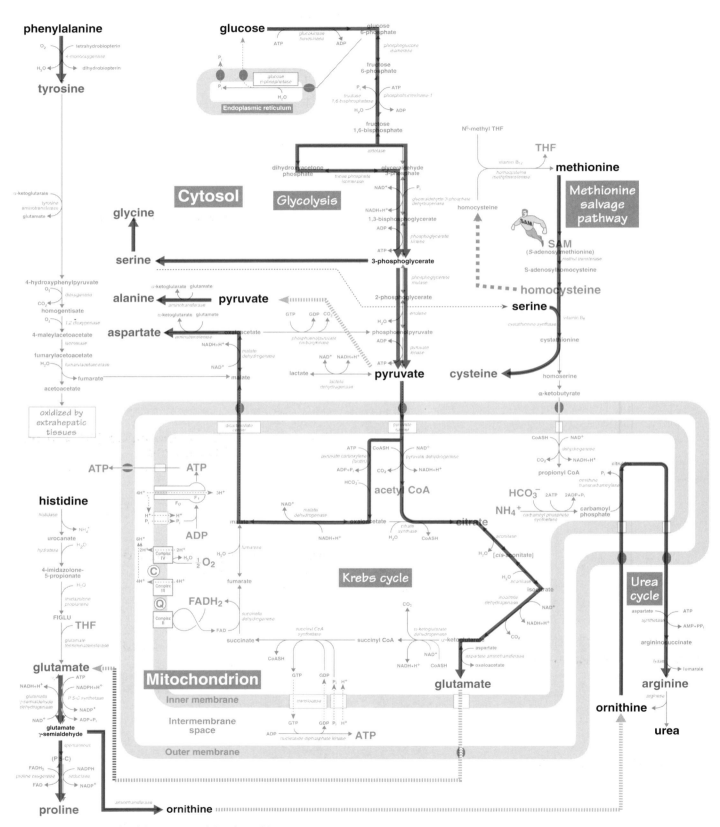

Figure 45.1 Biosynthesis of the non-essential amino acids.

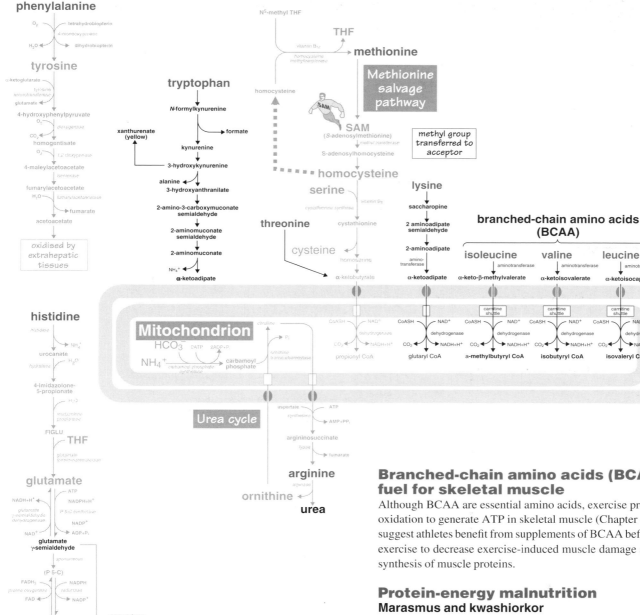

Figure 45.2 Overview of the catabolism of the essential amino acids.

Non-essential amino acids

Plants can make all the amino acids they need. However, animals (including humans) can synthesise only half the amino acids needed, namely Tyr, Gly, Ser, Ala, Asp, Cys, Glu, Pro, (Fig. 45.1). These are described as **non-essential amino acids**.

Essential amino acids

Humans cannot synthesise **P**he, **V**al, **T**ry, **T**hr, **I**so, **M**et, **H**is, **A**rg, **L**eu and **L**ys (*although it is generally thought that Arg and His are only needed by children during growth periods*). Catabolism of the essential amino acids are shown in Fig. 45.2.

Branched-chain amino acids (BCAA) as fuel for skeletal muscle

Although BCAA are essential amino acids, exercise promotes their oxidation to generate ATP in skeletal muscle (Chapter 46). Reports suggest athletes benefit from supplements of BCAA before and after exercise to decrease exercise-induced muscle damage and enhance synthesis of muscle proteins.

Protein-energy malnutrition
Marasmus and kwashiorkor

Marasmus is a term used for severe protein-energy malnutrition in children where the patient's weight is compared with an age-matched reference weight. Classifications vary but **normal nutrition is 90–110%** of reference weight. **Mild malnutrition is 75–90% and severe malnutrition (marasmus) is less than 60%** of reference weight matched for age.

If **oedema** is present, the malnutrition is termed **kwashiorkor** or **marasmus–kwashiorkor** if very severe.

Protein-energy malnutrition is very common in hospitalised patients, especially in the elderly and causes difficulties with wound healing and increased pressure sore development.

Cachexia

Cachexia is a term for extreme systemic atrophy. It generally occurs in adults where lack of nutrition causes atrophy of adipose tissue, the gut, pancreas and muscle. Cachexia is usually associated with the late stages of severe illness, especially cancer.

Amino acid metabolism: to energy as ATP; to glucose and ketone bodies

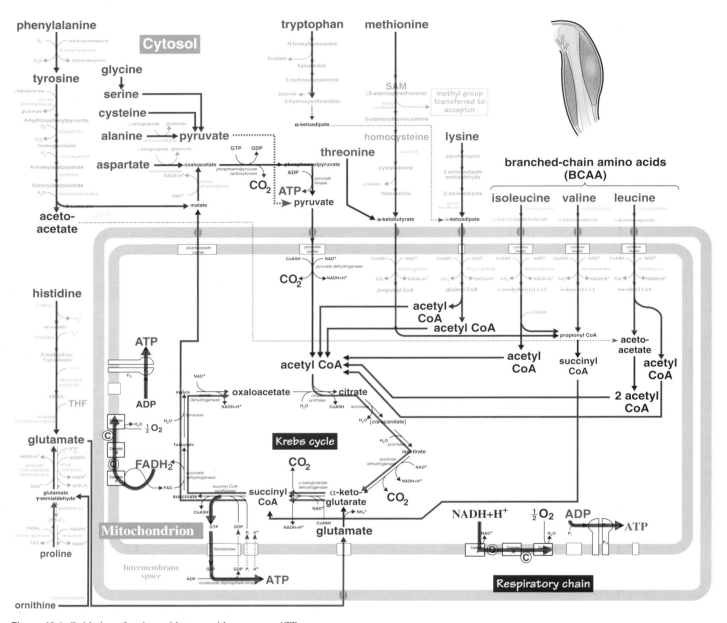

Figure 46.1 Oxidation of amino acids to provide energy as ATP.

Degradation of amino acids to provide energy as ATP

It is a common error perpetuated by most text books that the carbon "skeletons" derived from amino acids are oxidised when they enter Krebs cycle. **Note, that it is acetyl CoA that is oxidised to 2 molecules of CO₂.** Therefore, **before the amino acids can be fully oxidised they must be metabolised to acetyl CoA.** This is illustrated in

Fig. 46.1 where the majority of amino acids enter Krebs cycle directly as acetyl CoA for oxidation to produce NADH and FADH₂, which generate ATP in the respiratory chain. *NB Certain amino acids, namely **histidine**, **glutamate**, **proline**, and **ornithine** enter Krebs cycle as α-ketoglutarate, which is **partially** oxidised to form CO₂ by α-ketoglutarate dehydrogenase. However, the remainder of the "skeleton" must leave the mitochondrion for metabolism to **acetyl CoA** prior to complete oxidation.*

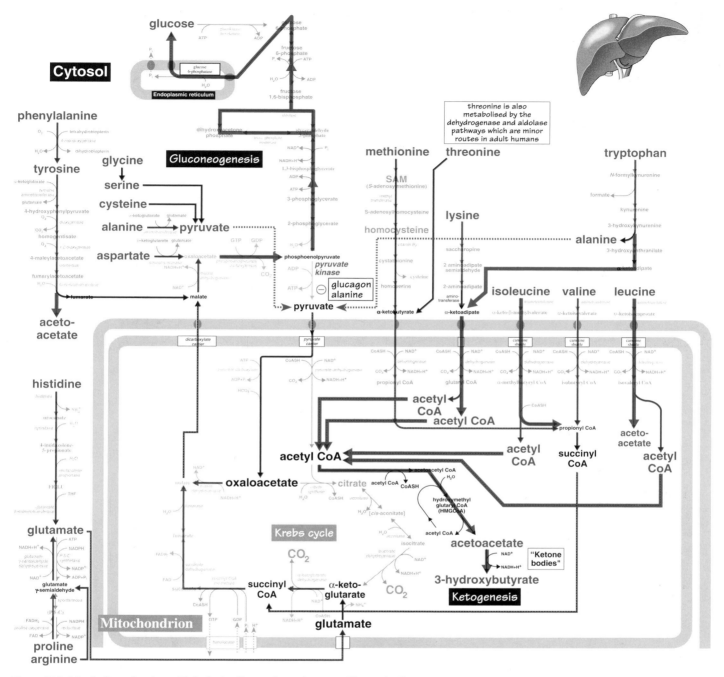

Figure 46.2 Metabolism of amino acids in fasting liver to form glucose and ketone bodies.

Metabolism of amino acids to glucose and/or ketone bodies

This is summarised in Fig. 46.2.

Glucogenic amino acids Glycine, serine, cysteine, alanine, aspartate, histidine, glutamate, proline, arginine, methionine, threonine and valine are glucogenic.

Ketogenic amino acids Lysine and leucine are ketogenic.

Amino acids that are both glucogenic and ketogenic Phenylalanine, tyrosine, isoleucine and tryptophan produce intermediates that can be metabolised to both glucose and the ketone bodies.

47
Amino acid disorders: maple syrup urine disease, homocystinuria, cystinuria, alkaptonuria and albinism

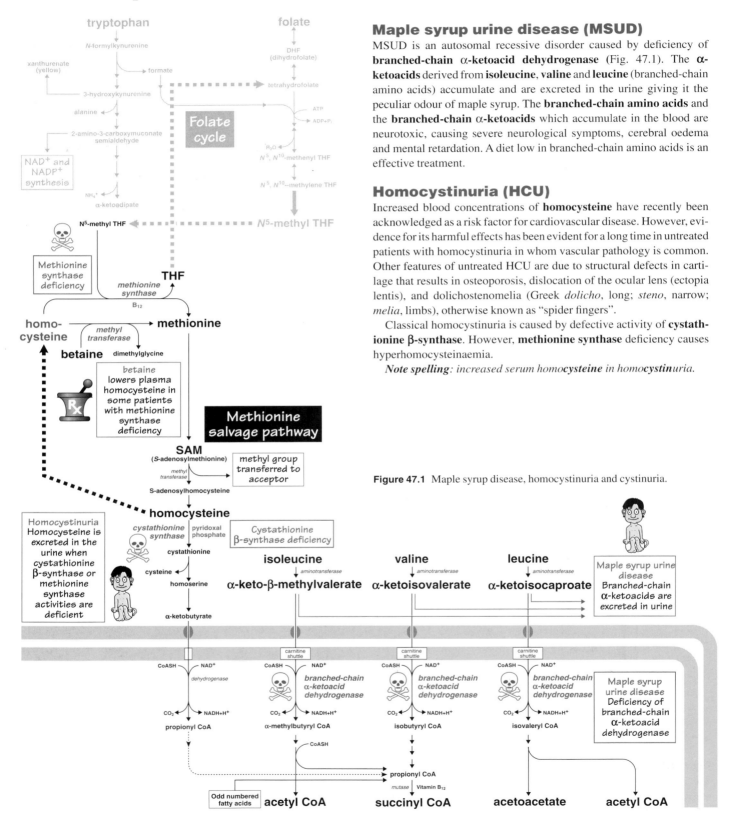

Maple syrup urine disease (MSUD)

MSUD is an autosomal recessive disorder caused by deficiency of **branched-chain α-ketoacid dehydrogenase** (Fig. 47.1). The **α-ketoacids** derived from **isoleucine**, **valine** and **leucine** (branched-chain amino acids) accumulate and are excreted in the urine giving it the peculiar odour of maple syrup. The **branched-chain amino acids** and the **branched-chain α-ketoacids** which accumulate in the blood are neurotoxic, causing severe neurological symptoms, cerebral oedema and mental retardation. A diet low in branched-chain amino acids is an effective treatment.

Homocystinuria (HCU)

Increased blood concentrations of **homocysteine** have recently been acknowledged as a risk factor for cardiovascular disease. However, evidence for its harmful effects has been evident for a long time in untreated patients with homocystinuria in whom vascular pathology is common. Other features of untreated HCU are due to structural defects in cartilage that results in osteoporosis, dislocation of the ocular lens (ectopia lentis), and dolichostenomelia (Greek *dolicho*, long; *steno*, narrow; *melia*, limbs), otherwise known as "spider fingers".

Classical homocystinuria is caused by defective activity of **cystathionine β-synthase**. However, **methionine synthase** deficiency causes hyperhomocysteinaemia.

*Note spelling: increased serum homo**cysteine** in homo**cystin**uria.*

Figure 47.1 Maple syrup disease, homocystinuria and cystinuria.

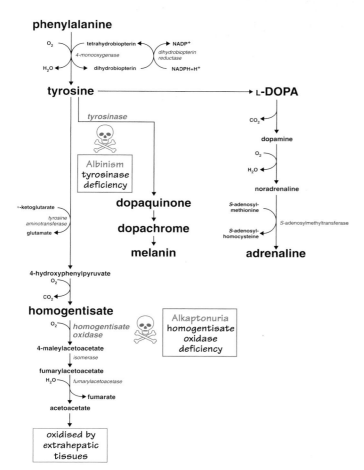

Figure 47.2 Albinism and alkaptonuria.

mulates in the tubular fluid, forming bladder and kidney stones (**cystine urolithiasis**). Cystine is so called because cystine stones were discovered in the cyst (i.e. bladder).

Alkaptonuria

Alkaptonuria is an autosomal recessive, benign disorder with a normal life expectancy. It is caused by a deficiency of **homogentisate oxidase** (Fig. 47.2). **Homogentisate** accumulates, is excreted in the urine and is gradually oxidised to a black pigment when exposed to air. It is usually detected when the nappies (or diapers) show **black staining**.

In the fourth decade signs of pigment staining appear (**onchrosis**) with slate blue or grey colouring of the ear cartilage.

Albinism (oculocutaneous albinism)

Albinism is a disorder of the synthesis or processing of the skin pigment, **melanin** (Fig. 47.2). **Oculocutaneous albinism type 1 (OCA type 1)** is an autosomal recessive disorder of **tyrosinase** resulting in the complete absence of pigment from the hair, eyes and skin. The lack of melanin in the skin makes OCA type 1 patients vulnerable to skin cancer.

Methionine synthase deficiency

Methionine synthase is a vitamin B_{12} dependent enzyme that needs N^5-**methyl THF** as a coenzyme (Fig. 47.1). It catalyses the transfer of the methyl group from N^5-methyl THF to **homocysteine** to form **methionine**. When methionine synthase activity is deficient homocysteine accumulates, causing hyperhomocystinaemia, megaloblastic anaemia and delayed development. Some patients with methionine synthase deficiency respond to supplementation with folate and vitamin B_{12}. Additional therapy using **betaine** exploits a shunt pathway that donates a methyl group to homocysteine, forming methionine.

Cystathionine β-synthase (CBS) deficiency

Cystathionine β-synthase deficiency is an autosomal recessive trait (Fig. 47.1). It is the most common cause of homocystinuria and is the second most treatable disorder of amino acid metabolism. Some patients respond to pyridoxine treatment but others are pyridoxine nonresponsive. Orally administered **betaine** often lowers serum homocysteine concentrations.

Cystinuria

Cystinuria is an autosomal recessive disorder of renal tubular reabsorption of **c**ystine, **o**rnithine, **a**rginine and **l**ysine (mnemonic: **COAL**). **Cystine** (a dimer of **cysteine**, Chapter 6), is sparingly soluble and accu-

48 Phenylalanine and tyrosine metabolism in health and disease

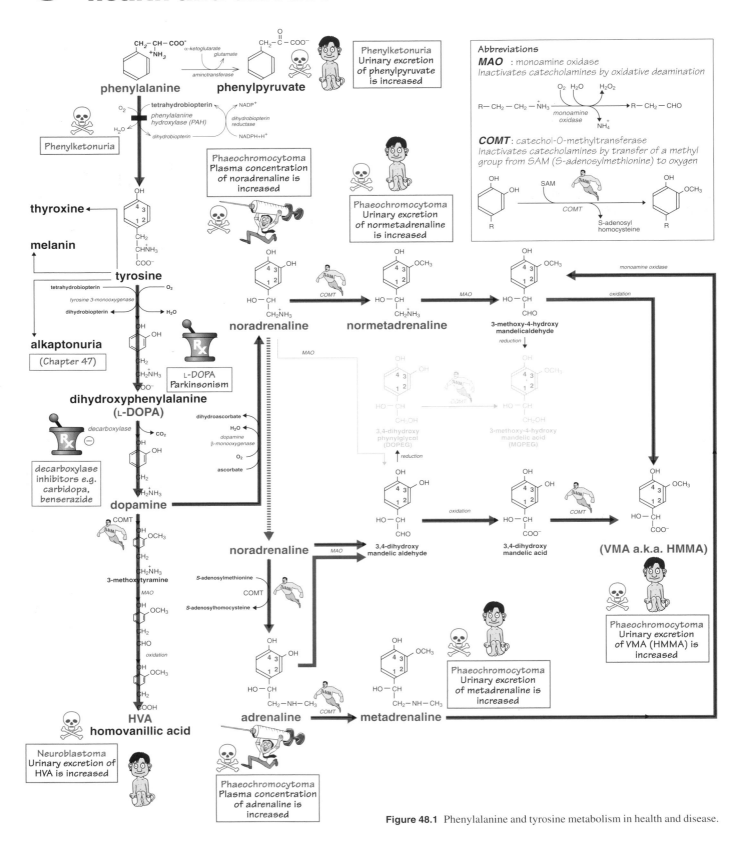

Figure 48.1 Phenylalanine and tyrosine metabolism in health and disease.

Metabolism of phenylalanine and tyrosine in health

Phenylalanine is an essential amino acid which can be oxidised at position 4 of the aromatic ring by **phenylalanine hydroxylase (PAH)** to form **tyrosine**. PAH (also known as phenylalanine 4-mono-oxygenase), needs **tetrahydrobiopterin (BH$_4$)** as a co-factor. Tyrosine is a precursor of the catecholamine hormones: **dopamine**, **noradrenaline** and **adrenaline**; and also the thyroid hormone **thyroxine**. **Adrenaline** (the English name from the Latin roots which describes its anatomical relationship to the "*kidney*") has been named in their spirit of independence by our American cousins as **epinephrine** from the Greek roots meaning "*above the kidney*". The name derives from its secretion by the medulla of the adrenal gland (which is situated above the kidney) and awaits renaming by the New World as the "epinephral" gland!

Metabolism of phenylalanine in disease: Phenylketonuria (PKU)

PKU is a genetic disorder characterised by deficient metabolism of phenylalanine, which results in the accumulation of phenylalanine and of the ketone, phenylpyruvate. Neonatal screening (recently improved by the introduction of tandem mass spectrometry) for PKU assists diagnosis and treatment, which minimises the mental retardation associated with this disorder. Classic PKU is an autosomal recessive disease due to deficient activity of PAH and needs treatment with a low phenylalanine diet. However, some patients lower their blood phenylalanine in response to a tetrahydrobiopterin (**BH$_4$**) loading test, particularly if the pure 6R-**BH$_4$** diastereoisomer is used.

Metabolism of tyrosine in disease: Alkaptonuria and albinism

These disorders of tyrosine metabolism are described in Chapter 47.

Metabolism of dopamine, noradrenaline and adrenaline

Biosynthesis

Tyrosine is the precursor of the **catecholamines** dopamine, noradrenaline and adrenaline. **Adrenaline** is stored in the chromaffin cells of the adrenal medulla and is secreted in the "fight or flight" response to danger. **Noradrenaline** (the "nor" prefix means it is adrenaline without the methyl group) is a neurotransmitter which is secreted into the synaptic cleft at nerve endings. **Dopamine**, which is an intermediate in the biosynthesis of noradrenaline and adrenaline, is localised in dopaminergic neurones, notably in the substantia nigra region of the brain.

Catabolism

The major enzymes in catecholamine catabolism are **catechol-O-methyltransferase (COMT)** and **monoamine oxidase (MAO)**. COMT transfers a **methyl** group from S-adenosylmethionine (**SAM**) (Chapter 47) to the **o**xygen at position 3 of the aromatic ring (Fig. 48.1). The pathway taken is a lottery depending whether the noradrenaline and adrenaline are first of all **methylated** (by **COMT**) or alternatively **oxidatively deaminated** (by **MAO**). If chance determines methylation has priority, then the "methylated amines" **normetadrenaline** and **metadrenaline** are formed prior to the MAO reaction and subsequent oxidation to **HMMA** (also known as **vanillylmandelic acid (VMA)** or **3-methoxy-4-hydroxymandelic acid (MHMA)**). On the other hand, if fate determines that the MAO reaction occurs first, then oxidation followed by methylation by COMT is the route taken to HMMA.

Catecholamine metabolism in disease

Dopamine deficiency in Parkinson's disease

In this "shaking palsy" as it was first described in 1817, the dopamine-containing neurones in the substantia nigra region of the brain degenerate. Dosing with **L-DOPA**, which crosses the **blood–brain barrier (BBB)** and is a precursor of **dopamine** (which cannot cross the BBB), provided a dramatic breakthrough in treatment. This was refined by combination with drugs such as **carbidopa** and **benserazide** (which cannot cross the BBB) as they inhibit the wasteful catabolism of L-DOPA by peripheral **decarboxylase** activity enabling much smaller doses of L-DOPA to be used as a precursor for dopamine in the brain.

Excessive production of adrenaline in phaeochromocytoma

A phaeochromocytoma is a rare tumour of the adrenal medulla that produces large amounts of adrenaline and/or noradrenaline. Until the 1990s they were frequently overlooked and most cases were diagnosed *post mortem*. Nowadays, abdominal MRI scans reveal the tumours which can be removed by surgery. Patients suffer episodes of severe hypertension, sweating and headaches. The episodic nature of this condition means that blood and urine samples for laboratory analysis should be collected immediately after an attack as the results of tests collected between episodes are frequently normal. Laboratory investigations are urine collections for **metadrenaline**, **normetadrenaline** and **HMMA**. Sometimes, it is useful to measure blood levels of **adrenaline** and **noradrenaline**.

Excessive production of dopamine

Neuroblastomas produce large amounts of dopamine anywhere in the body. They usually occur in children under 5 years old and are of neural crest cell origin. Biochemical markers are **HMMA** and the dopamine catabolic product **homovanillic acid (HVA)**.

49 The products of tryptophan and histidine metabolism

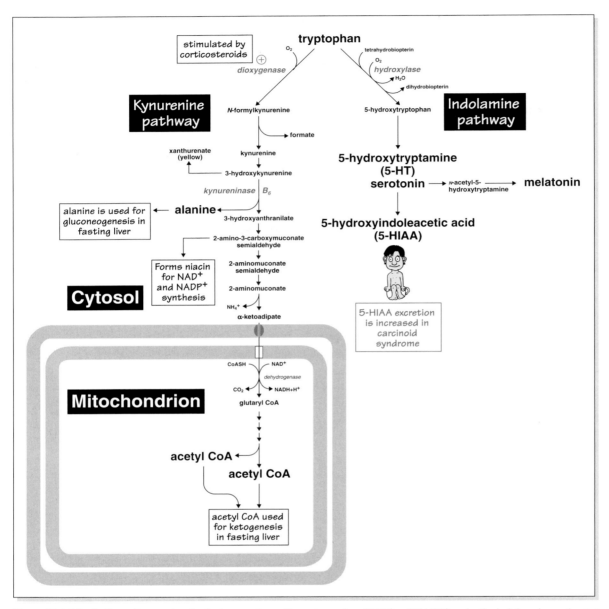

Figure 49.1 Metabolism of tryptophan by the kynurenine pathway to produce NAD^+ and $NADP^+$; or by the indoleamine pathway to produce serotonin and melatonin.

Tryptophan is the precursor of NAD^+, $NADP^+$, serotonin and melatonin

The production of NAD^+ and $NADP^+$ by the kynurenine pathway

The **kynurenine pathway** (Fig. 49.1) is the principal pathway for tryptophan metabolism and it produces precursors which, together with dietary niacin, are used to synthesise NAD^+ and $NADP^+$ (Chapter 55). It is generally accepted that 60 mg of tryptophan is equivalent to 1 mg of niacin.

Serotonin

Serotonin (5-hydroxytryptamine) is produced from tryptophan by the **indoleamine pathway**. Serotonin is important for a feeling of well-being and a deficiency of brain serotonin is associated with depression. The **selective serotonin re-uptake inhibitors (SSRIs)** are a successful class of antidepressive drugs that prolong the presence of serotonin in the synaptic cleft thereby stimulating synaptic transmission in neurones which produce a sense of euphoria.

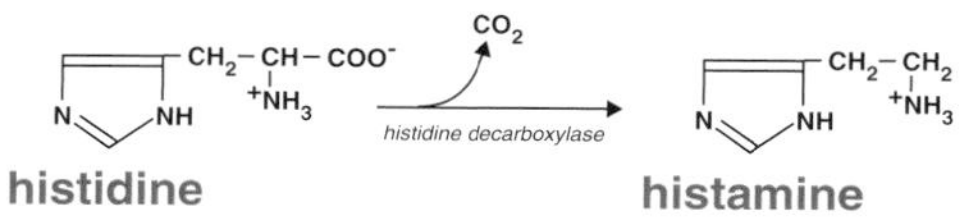

Figure 49.2 Production of histamine from histidine.

Monoamine hypothesis of depression

The "monoamine hypothesis of depression" was proposed over 35 years ago to describe the biochemical lesion in depression. Basically, it proposes that **depression** is caused by **depletion** of monoamines (e.g. **noradrenaline** and or **serotonin**) from the synapses which reduces synaptic activity in the brain causing **depression**. Conversely, it suggests that **mania** is caused by an **excess** of monoamines in synapses, with excessive synaptic activity in the brain resulting in **excessive euphoria**.

There is evidence that systemic **corticosteroids lower serotonin** levels. This is because corticosteroids stimulate the activity of **dioxygenase**, which increases the flow of tryptophan metabolites along the kynurenine pathway at the expense of the **indoleamine pathway** and the production of serotonin. Lower brain concentrations of serotonin may be associated with depression. Patients with high cortisol levels (e.g. in Cushing's syndrome) are depressed which is consistent with this hypothesis.

Carcinoid syndrome and 5-HIAA

Serotonin is metabolised to **5-hydroxyindoleacetic acid (5-HIAA)** which is excreted in the urine. Patients with carcinoid syndrome excrete increased amounts of 5-HIAA.

Melatonin

Melatonin is made in the pineal gland and is secreted during periods of darkness. Typically, melatonin secretion begins at night-time when it aids sleeping. During daylight hours, the blood concentration of melatonin is very low.

Histamine

Histamine is involved in local immune responses and in allergenic reactions. It is also involved in controlling the amount of gastric acid produced. Histamine is produce from histidine by a decarboxylation reaction (Fig. 49.2).

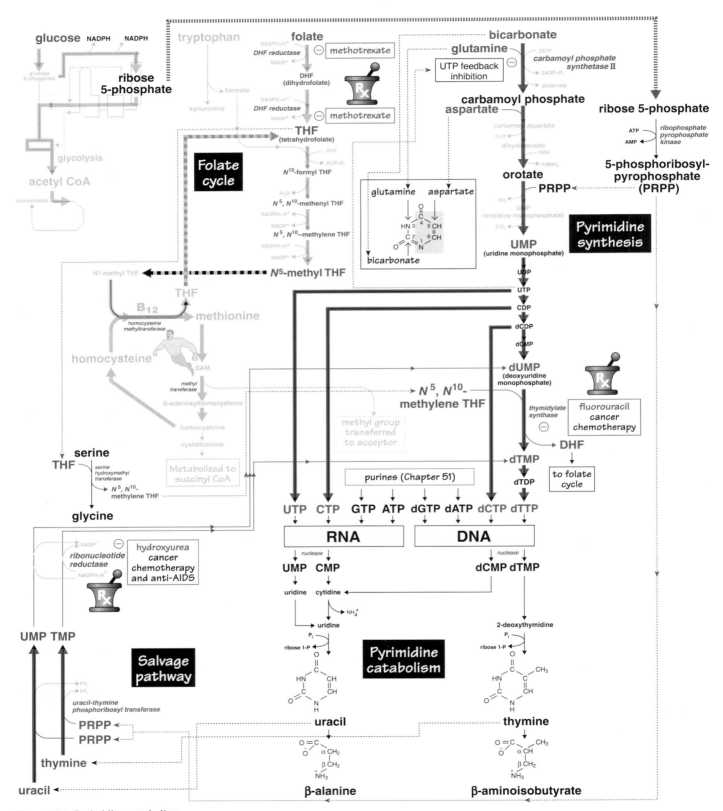

Figure 50.1 Pyrimidine metabolism.

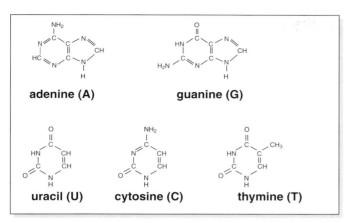

Figure 50.2 Purine and pyrimidine bases.

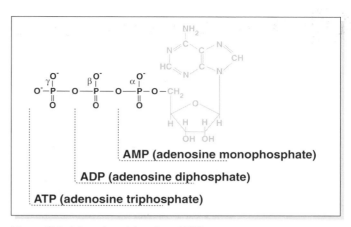

Figure 50.3 Adenosine triphosphate (ATP).

Bases, nucleoside and nucleotides

The **purine bases** are **adenine** (A) and **guanine** (G). **The pyrimidine bases** are **cytosine** (C), **thymine** (T) and **uracil** (U) (Fig. 50.2).

The bases combine with ribose or deoxyribose (e.g. dUMP) to form their corresponding **nucleosides: adenosine, guanosine, cytidine, thymidine** and **uridine**.

The addition of one or more phosphates forms the corresponding **nucleotide**, e.g. adenosine (the nucleoside) can form the nucleotides: adenosine monophosphate (AMP), adenosine diphosphate (ADP) and **adenosine triphosphate (ATP)** (Fig. 50.3).

NB When the bases occur in nucleic acids, adenine, guanine and cytosine are present in both RNA and DNA; uracil is found only in RNA; and thymine is found only in DNA. (*Attention: do not confuse "thymine" with vitamin B$_1$ which is "thiamin".*)

Pyrimidines and purines are important for cell growth and division

The pyrimidines and purines have many roles as substrates, coenzymes and signalling molecules and as such play numerous important roles in metabolism. Also, they are major components of DNA and RNA. Accordingly, they are vital for cell growth and division. Not surprisingly, the development and growth of the foetus *in utero* demands a substantial supply of purines and pyrimidines and it is important that the substrates and co-factors needed for their biosynthesis are available to the mother at conception and throughout pregnancy. There is a particular need for **vitamin B$_{12}$** and **folate** (Chapter 57) and deficiency of these vitamins is associated with birth defects. On the other hand, when an ectopic pregnancy must be terminated, treatment with **methotrexate** (a folate antagonist, see below) has been advocated recently.

Biosynthesis of pyrimidines

The precursors of the pyrimidine ring are **bicarbonate, glutamine** and **aspartate** (Fig. 50.1). The regulatory enzyme is **carbamoylphosphate synthetase II (CPS II)** which is subject to feedback inhibition by uridine triphosphate (UTP). NB CPS II is different from **CPS I** which provides carbamoyl phosphate for, and is the regulatory enzyme of, the urea cycle (Chapter 44). They differ in that CPS I is a **mitochondrial**

enzyme that obtains nitrogen from **ammonia**, while CPS II is **cytosolic** and obtains its nitrogen from the γ-amide of **glutamine**. Another precursor that is needed to methylate **dUMP** to form **dTMP**, is N^5,N^{10}-**methylene THF**. dTTP is essential for DNA biosynthesis.

Catabolism of pyrimidines

CMP and **dCMP** are deaminated to **uracil** and **dTMP** is degraded to **thymine**. Both uracil and thymine can be recycled to nucleotides by the **salvage pathway**. Alternatively, they can be degraded to **β-alanine** and **β-aminoisobutyrate**, respectively.

Cancer chemotherapy

Cancer cells divide and grow much more rapidly than normal cells and have a great need for DNA and RNA synthesis during the **S** phase (synthetic) of the "cell cycle". This provides a strategy for devising anti-cancer drugs and so folate antagonists, anti-pyrimidines and anti-purines (known as anti-metabolites) which inhibit cell proliferation, have been developed.

Folate antagonist

Methotrexate is a close structural analogue of folate and inhibits **dihydrofolate reductase**. This prevents the reduction of folate and dihydrofolate (**DHF**) to tetrahydrofolate (**THF**) which is the precursor of N^5,N^{10}-methylene THF. This is essential for dTTP and DNA synthesis. Unfortunately, normal cells are also attacked by methotrexate. Folinic acid (N^5-formyl tetrahydrofolate) is an active form of folate that can be given after the start of methotrexate treatment to rescue normal cells from this drug toxicity.

Antipyrimidines

Anti-cancer drugs based on pyrimidine analogues containing fluorine (the fluoropyrimidines, e.g. **5-fluorouracil** (5-FU)) have been used successfully to treat cancer. 5-FU acts by inhibiting **thymidylate synthase** thus preventing the methylation of **dUMP** to **dTMP** which is a vital precursor for DNA biosynthesis.

Antipurines

Purine antimetabolites are described in Chapter 51.

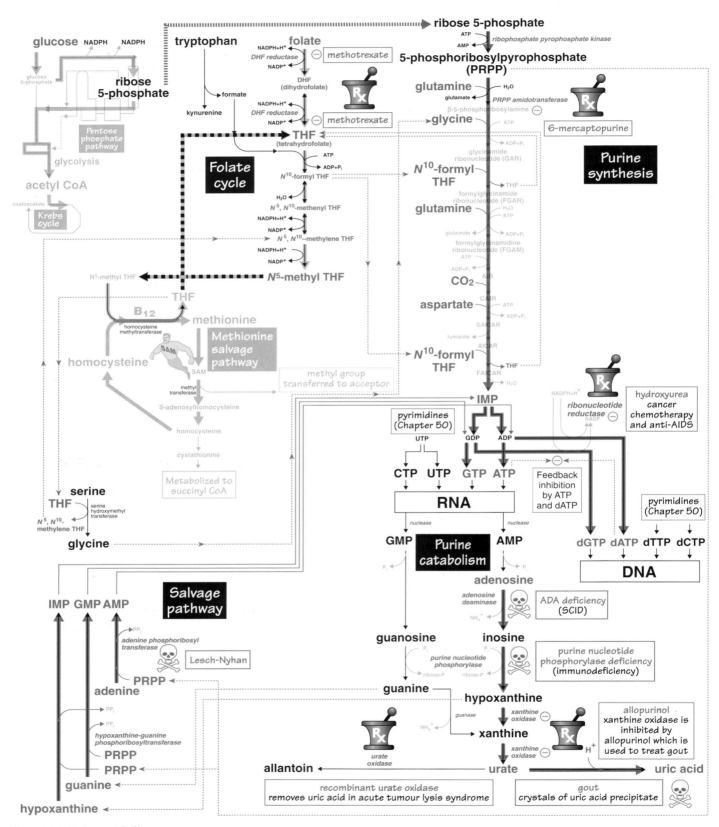

Figure 51.1 Purine metabolism.

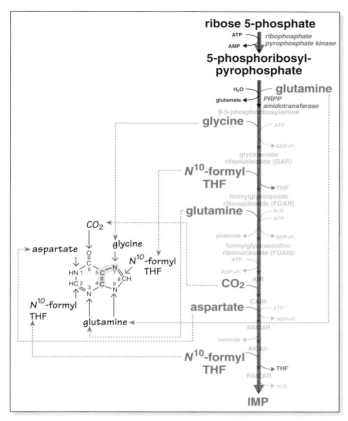

Figure 51.2 The origin of the atoms in the purine molecule.

Biosynthesis and breakdown of purines

The purine nucleotides GTP and ATP are very important in intermediary metabolism and the regulation of metabolism. Adenine is also a component of cyclic AMP, FAD, NAD$^+$, NADP$^+$ and coenzyme A. Moreover, GTP, ATP and their deoxy-derivatives dGTP and dATP are important precursors for the synthesis of RNA and DNA, which are essential for cell growth and division. **Purine biosynthesis** (Fig. 51.1) needs the amino acids **glutamine**, **glycine** and **aspartate**. Also, **tryptophan** is needed to supply formate which reacts with tetrahydrofolate (THF) to produce N^{10}-**formyl THF**, which donates the **formyl** group to the purine structure. A molecule of CO_2 is also needed.

Purine catabolism produces **urate**, which has the disadvantage of being sparingly soluble in the aqueous environment of blood and has a tendency to precipitate as **uric acid**, with the pathological consequences (gout) described below.

Origin of the atoms in the purine molecule

The origin of the atoms in the purine molecule is shown in Fig. 51.2.

Cancer chemotherapy

Methotrexate, **6-mercaptopurine** and **hydroxyurea** all inhibit the synthesis of purine nucleotides or purine deoxynucleotides. These respectively are essential components of RNA and DNA which are vital for cell division and growth. Cancer cells which are dividing and growing rapidly compared with healthy cells e.g. high grade lymphomas, are particularly vulnerable to these drugs.

Adenosine deaminase deficiency and severe combined immunodeficiency (SCID)

Adenosine deaminase deficiency (ADA deficiency) is a very rare autosomal recessive disease and is responsible for 20–30% of recessively inherited cases of SCID. It causes ATP and dATP to accumulate which feed-back to inhibit ribonucleotide reductase in thymocytes and peripheral blood B cells. This in turn restricts the formation of DNA and hence the production of T and B cells (SCID). Infants are extremely vulnerable to infection as exemplified by the case in the 1970s of David Vetter who spent his entire life of 12 years protected inside a plastic bubble and is immortalised in the film *The Boy in the Plastic Bubble*. Clinical trials of gene therapy for ADA-SCID are encouraging.

Gout

Gout is commonly associated with rich food and alcohol consumption. Rich food is a source of dietary DNA and RNA, which is broken down to urate. Alcohol causes accumulation of lactate, which competes with urate for excretion by the kidney. Gout results when the concentration of urate (which is sparingly soluble) in the blood increases to a concentration when it is precipitated as crystals of uric acid. This causes considerable pain as illustrated in the picture *The Gout* by James Gilray in 1799. The needle-shaped crystals of uric acid can be deposited around joints, especially in the big toe. Crystals can also be deposited in the urinary tract as renal stones or in the skin as tophi, e.g. in the ear lobe. Gout is treated with the xanthine oxidase inhibitor, allopurinol, which restricts the production of uric acid.

Acute tumour lysis syndrome (ATLS)

ATLS is potentially a catastrophic complication of chemotherapy in patients with a high tumour load. It results from cytotoxic damage to large numbers of cancerous cells. The DNA and RNA released are broken down to uric acid which precipitates in the renal tubules causing acute uric acid nephropathy. Recent evidence suggests that **recombinant urate oxidase**, which converts uric acid to soluble allantoin, is successful in the treatment and prevention of ATLS in patients with haematological malignancies.

Lesch-Nyhan syndrome (LNS)

LNS is a rare, X-linked disorder of **adenine phosphoribosyl transferase** in the purine salvage pathway. This causes severe accumulation of uric acid resulting in gout and renal stones. The condition is characterised by mental retardation and compulsive self-mutilation with biting of the lips, tongue and fingers and head banging.

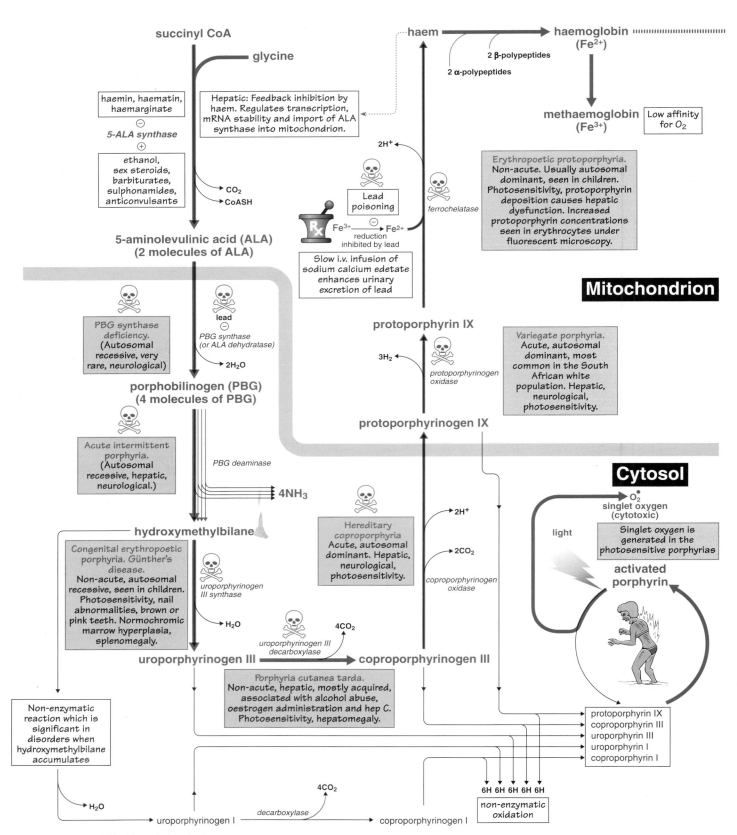

Figure 52.1 Haem, bilirubin and phorphyria.

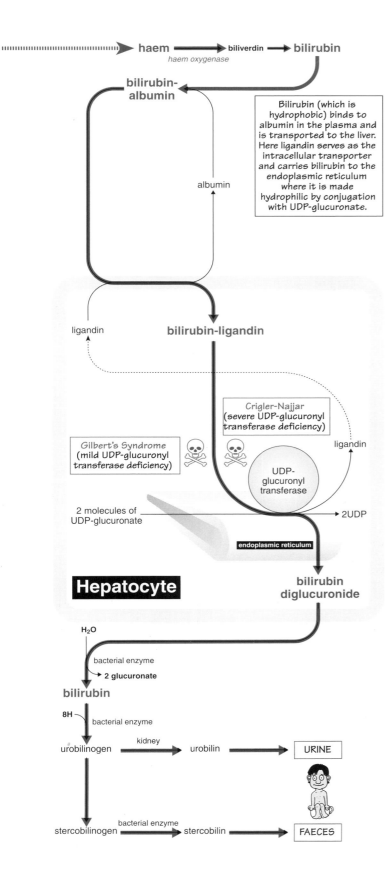

Haem biosynthesis

Haem is synthesised from **succinyl CoA** and **glycine** in most cells but particularly in liver and the haemopoietic cells of bone marrow. Hepatic haem is used to produce several haem proteins especially the cytochrome P_{450} (CYP) family of enzymes and respiratory chain cytochromes In erythrocytes, haem combines with globin to form haemoglobin. Haem biosynthesis is regulated by **5-aminolevulinic acid synthase (5-ALA synthase)** which, in the liver, is controlled through feedback inhibition by haem. Hence, if the concentration of haem decreases, then 5-ALA synthase will be stimulated. The pathway also involves **porphobilinogen (PBG)**. PBG is deaminated to form **hydroxymethylbilane** which cyclises to **uroporphyrinogen III**, the precursor of haem (Fig. 52.1).

Acute intermittent porphyria (AIP)

This autosomal dominant condition is caused by deficiency of **PBG deaminase** and, unlike the other porphyrias, does not cause photosensitivity. The acute gastrointestinal and neuropsychiatric symptoms of AIP are caused by accumulation of 5-ALA and PBG. Episodes are triggered by ingesting alcohol and a variety of drugs, e.g. barbiturates and oral contraceptives. This is because these agents are metabolised by the cytochrome P_{450} system. Since haem is a component of cytochrome P_{450}, induction of these enzymes incorporates the available haem, consequently the haem concentration falls, the negative feedback to 5-ALA synthase is reduced and so production of PBG is enhanced. Unfortunately, because of PBG deaminase deficiency, this induced surge in **PBG accumulates** and provokes the symptoms of AIP. In AIP patients, the **urine** turns the colour of **port wine** on standing. Diagnosis is confirmed by **urine PBG excretion**. Treatment is directed at reducing 5-ALA synthase activity by i.v. infusion of haematin.

The photosensitive porphyrias

The deficiency of enzymes downstream of **hydroxymethylbilane** cause accumulation of intermediates which are diverted by non-enzymic oxidation to form several porphyrins which, when exposed to light, form **singlet oxygen $O_2^{\cdot}$**. This is cytotoxic, causing photosensitivity on exposure to sunlight.

Lead poisoning

Lead inhibits **PBG synthase** and **ferrochelatase**, restricting haem biosynthesis and resulting in microcytic hypochromic anaemia and porphyria. Urinary excretion of 5-ALA is increased.

Haem catabolism to bilirubin

Haem is degraded by **haem oxygenase** in the reticuloendothelial system to **bilirubin**. Bilirubin is hydrophobic and is transported in the blood by albumin. In jaundice, bilirubin is produced in excess and the lipophilic bilirubin accumulates in the brain causing kernicterus. Normally, bilirubin is conjugated in the liver to **bilirubin diglucuronide** which is water soluble and is excreted in the bile. Bilirubin diglucuronide then passes into the small intestine where bacterial enzymes produce **urobilinogen**. Urobilinogen can be absorbed and passed to the liver where it is re-excreted in the bile. A small amount, however, is excreted in urine as **urobilin**. Urobilinogen remaining in the intestine is converted to **stercobilin** which is egested in the faeces.

53

Fat-soluble vitamins I: vitamins A and D

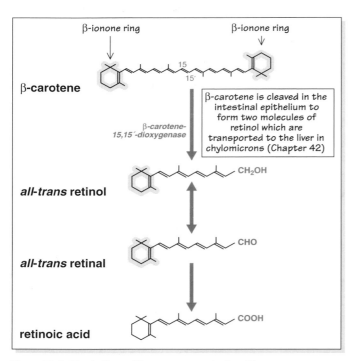

Figure 53.1 Metabolism of β-carotene to retinoic acid.

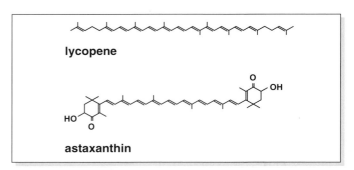

Figure 53.2 Lycopene and astaxanthin are carotenoids (but not vitamin A precursors).

The fat-soluble vitamins A, D, E and K, are absorbed by the intestines and incorporated into chylomicrons (Chapter 42). Therefore, diseases which affect fat absorption causing steatorrhoea will also affect the uptake of these vitamins. Furthermore, fat absorption relies on pancreatic lipase which if compromised, e.g. in cystic fibrosis, can cause deficiency of one or more fat-soluble vitamins.

Vitamin A

Vitamin A is a generic term that includes "**preformed vitamin A**", namely "**retinol** (alcohol), **retinal** (aldehyde), and **retinoic acid** (carboxylic acid)"; and the **provitamin A carotenoids** which are those carotenoids capable of metabolism to retinol, e.g. β-**carotene** (Fig. 53.1).

Biochemical function

1. Vision. Retinol is metabolised to 11-*cis* retinal which binds to opsin in the rod cells forming the visual pigment "rhodopsin". A photon of light converts 11-*cis* retinal to *all-trans* retinal, initiating a series of reactions culminating in a signal to the optic nerve. This is transmitted to the brain where it is interpreted as a visual image.

2. Control of gene expression. Retinal can be oxidised to retinoic acid which affects gene expression. Inside the nucleus, retinoic acid binds to receptors that regulate the activity of chromosomal retinoic acid response elements (RARE). By stimulating and repressing gene transcription, retinoic acid regulates the differentiation of cells and so is important for growth and development, including lymphocytes which are vital for the immune response.

Deficiency diseases

1. Vision disorders. Early vitamin A deficiency causes impaired night vision. Severe vitamin A deficiency causes xerophthalmia which progresses to corneal scarring and blindness. It occurs in over 100 million children in poor nations where rice is the staple food.

2. Cell differentiation disorders. Vitamin A is the "anti-infection vitamin". Impaired cell differentiation caused by vitamin A deficiency impairs formation of lymphocytes and is manifest as immunodeficiency disease resulting in increased susceptibility to infectious diseases.

Dietary sources

Vitamin A is available either from: (i) **preformed retinol** (present in animal foods as retinyl esters), or (ii) metabolised from **provitamin A precursors**. The recommended dietary allowance for preformed vitamin A is 0.9 mg/day for men and 0.7 mg/day for women. Provitamin A sources are graded according to their **retinol activity equivalence (RAE),** e.g. since 12 mg of β-carotene in food yields 1 mg retinol, its RAE is 12.

1. Preformed vitamin A. Liver products, fortified breakfast cereals, eggs, dairy products.

2. Provitamin A. Carotenoids are a large family of coloured compounds that are abundant in plants. About 10% of carotenoids have the β-**ionone ring** which is needed for vitamin A activity, e.g. β-**carotene** found in carrots. Carotenoids have numerous double bonds which ensure they are efficient **free radical scavengers** and they can neutralise singlet oxygen.

Not all carotenoids are vitamin A precursors. These comprise 90% of carotenoids, nevertheless they are excellent free radical scavengers. Examples are **lycopene** (in tomatoes) and **astaxanthin** (Fig. 53.2). The latter is enjoying a reputation as a nutriceutical. It is pink and found in aquatic animals, e.g. salmon, shrimp, lobster and in the alga, *Haematococcus pluvialis*, from which it is commercially extracted.

Toxicity

Hypervitaminosis A results from excessive intake of preformed vitamin A. Toxicity in pregnancy is related to the role of retinoic acid in regulating differentiation, resulting in birth defects. Recent reports suggest that habitual high doses of vitamin A might be associated with osteoporosis.

Polar bear liver is toxic! 500 g of polar bear liver contains up to 10 million IU of vitamin A. Arctic explorers, their dogs and Inuit people have suffered acute vitamin A toxicity after eating it.

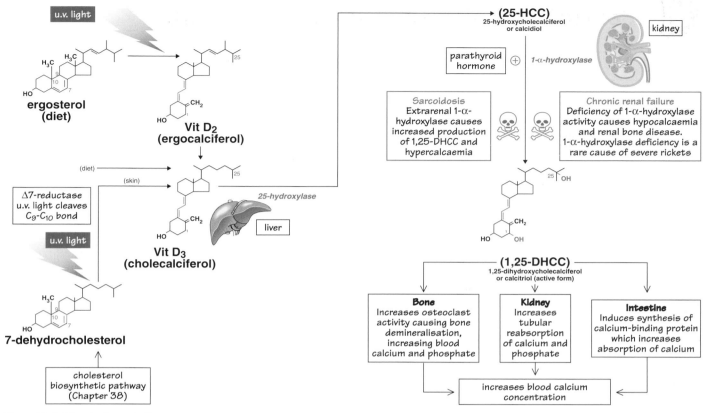

Figure 53.3 Vitamin D metabolism

Vitamin A analogues

Isotretinoin and etretinate are analogues of vitamin A used to treat skin disorders. Isotretinoin is used to treat severe acne (but must be avoided in pregnancy, see above). Etretinate was used to treat psoriasis but it has been withdrawn in some countries.

Vitamin D

Vitamin D is the "**sunshine vitamin**". It was originally discovered as a crude mixture called **vitamin D$_1$** (no longer available as a supplement). **Ergosterol**, the plant equivalent of cholesterol, is converted to **vitamin D$_2$** by ultraviolet light. **Vitamin D$_3$ (cholecalciferol)** is formed in the skin from **7-dehydrocholesterol**, (an intermediate in the cholesterol biosynthesis pathway) in the presence of ultraviolet light, which opens the B ring of the steroid nucleus (Fig. 53.3). Cholecalciferol is successively hydroxylated first in the liver forming 25-hydroxycholecalciferol (25-HCC) and then in the kidney to form the most active form: **1,25-dihydroxycholecalciferol (1,25-DHCC)**, also known as **calcitriol**.

Biochemical function

1,25-DHCC controls calcium metabolism by increasing blood calcium. It increases **intestinal** absorption of dietary calcium, in **bone** it stimulates resorption of calcium, and in **kidney** it stimulates reabsorption of calcium into the blood.

Diagnostic tests for deficiency

Urinary calcium is low. Measure serum 25-HCC.

Dietary sources

There are few natural dietary sources but these include fish liver oils and fatty fish (e.g. sardines, mackerel, salmon). Several foods e.g. breakfast cereals, orange juice, margarine and milk, are fortified with vitamin D (cholecalciferol or ergocalciferol).

Deficiency diseases

Deficiency causes hypocalcaemia, resulting in rickets in children or osteomalacia in adults. Hypocalcaemic convulsions and tetany can occur.

1. Lack of sunlight. Exposure to sunlight can provide sufficient vitamin D. However, in latitudes greater than 40° north or south "vitamin D winter deficiency" can occur. People with dark skin can suffer deficiency especially if their skin is completely covered and they live in the northern or southern latitudes previously mentioned. Such people, for example Muslim women living in northern Europe, can be hypocalcaemic.

2. Malabsorption. Steatorrhoea caused by exocrine pancreatic disease, or biliary obstruction can cause vitamin D deficiency.

3. Chronic renal failure. Normal kidney function is needed for the α-1 hydroxylation reaction that produces 1,25-DHCC. In chronic renal failure a cascade of events is triggered, leading to secondary hyperparathyroidism, which can progress to tertiary hyperparathyroidism and renal bone disease.

Toxicity

Hypervitaminosis D produces hypercalcaemia which can result in bone loss, organ calcification (e.g. kidneys and heart) and kidney stones.

Vitamin D hypersensitivity in sarcoidosis: extrarenal 1 α-hydroxylase activity occurs in sarcoid granulomas which converts vitamin D to inappropriately high concentrations of 1,25-DHCC, causing hypercalcaemia. Also occurs in some lymphomas and sarcomas.

54

Fat-soluble vitamins II: vitamins E and K

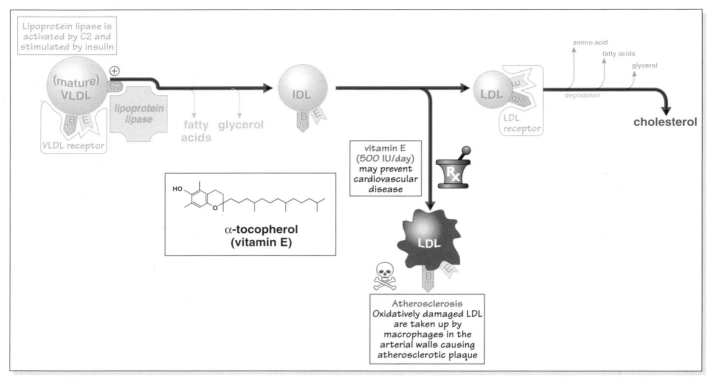

Figure 54.1 Vitamin E reduces oxidative damage to low density lipoproteins (LDLs).

Vitamin E

Vitamin E is a generic term for four tocopherols (α-, β-, γ- and δ-) and four tocotrienols (α-, β-, γ- and δ-). Of these, **α-tocopherol** is the most important.

Biochemical function

α-Tocopherol is an antioxidant that prevents free radical damage to polyunsaturated fatty acids, particularly those in the cell membrane of red blood cells. Evidence suggests α-**tocopherol** reduces oxidative damage to low density lipoproteins (LDLs) which is associated with the development of atherosclerosis (Chapters 19, 39). Disappointingly, claims that dietary supplementation with α-**tocopherol** decreases cardiovascular disease are controversial. However, recent studies using 500 IU α-**tocopherol**/day claim inhibition of lipid oxidation in atherosclerotic lesions.

Diagnostic test for deficiency

Measure platelet vitamin E concentration.

Dietary sources

Vegetable oils, nuts and green leafy vegetables.

Deficiency diseases

Occurs in children with cystic fibrosis and patients with steatorrhoea. Red cell membrane damage results in haemolytic anaemia. Damage to nerve cells causes peripheral neuropathy.

Toxicity

Few toxic effects have been reported, however high doses might cause increased clotting times in subjects with a low vitamin K status.

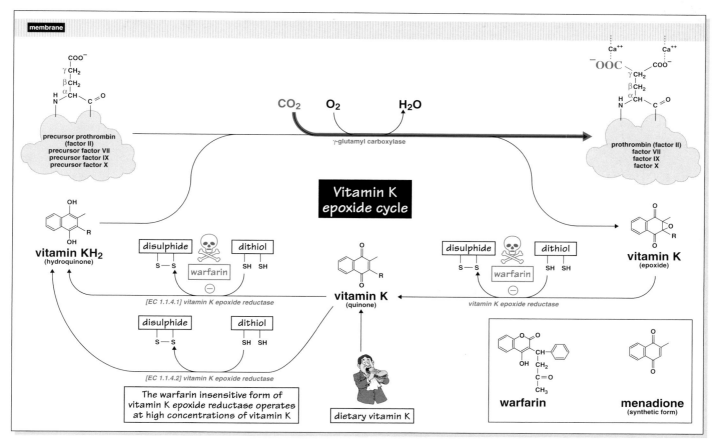

Figure 54.2 The vitamin K epoxide cycle.

Vitamin K

Vitamin K, from the Danish "Koagulation", exists in two natural forms: **vitamin K₁ (phylloquinone)**, and **vitamin K₂ (menaquinone)**. **Vitamin K₃ (menadione)** is a synthetic, water-soluble analogue.

Biochemical functions

Vitamin K is essential for activity of **vitamin K-dependent γ-glutamyl carboxylase** which is responsible for post-translational modification of glutamyl residues (Glu) to γ-carboxylated glutamyl residues (Gla) producing a small family of **"vitamin K- dependent proteins, VKD proteins**). It is membrane bound and carboxylates the proteins as they emerge from the endoplasmic reticulum. The VKD proteins associated with blood clotting are well established but recent research has revealed VKD proteins associated with bone metabolism (bone Gla protein (BGP) and matrix Gla protein (MGP)).

1. Blood clotting: The precursors of the **anticoagulants prothrombin and factors VII, IX** and **X** are activated when **glutamate** (Glu) residues are carboxylated to **γ-carboxyglutamate (Gla)** by a vitamin K-dependent reaction. This process is linked to regeneration of vitamin K in the **"vitamin K epoxide cycle"**.

2. Bone mineralisation. Recent evidence is emerging that suggests that vitamin K plays a role in bone growth and development.

Diagnostic test for deficiency

Measure undercarboxylated Gla proteins in blood.

Dietary sources

The major source is **phylloquinone (vitamin K₁)** found in vegetable oils and green leafy vegetables. **Menaquinone (vitamin K₂)** is synthesised by the flora of the large intestine.

Deficiency diseases

1. Haemorrhagic disease of the newborn Placental transfer of vitamin K is inefficient so deficiency can occur resulting in neonatal haemorrhage.

2. Newborns have a sterile intestinal tract and there is therefore no bacterial source.

3. Breast milk is a poor source of vitamin K.

4. Osteoporosis. Recent research has investigated an association between osteoporotic fracture and vitamin K.

Toxicity

Toxicity with high doses of phylloquinone and menaquinone has not been reported. However, i.v. menadione causes oxidative damage to red cell membranes (haemolysis).

55

Water-soluble vitamins I: thiamin, riboflavin, niacin and pantothenate

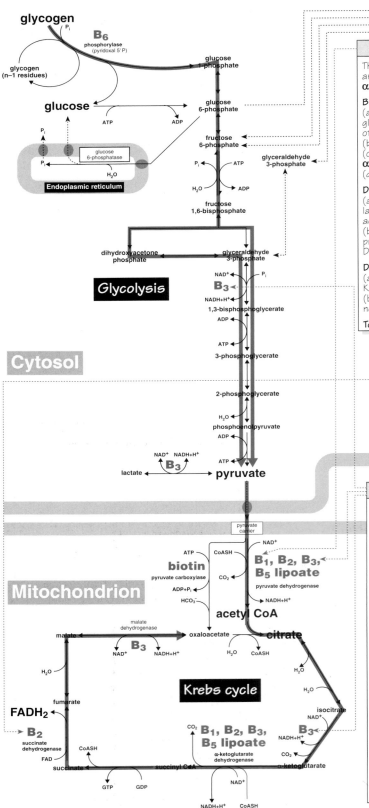

Thiamin pyrophosphate (Vitamin B₁)

Thiamin pyrophosphate (Vitamin B₁) is essential for pyruvate dehydrogenase and similar large multienzyme complexes which oxidatively decarboxylate α-ketoacids. RNI 0.4 mg/1000 Kcal (depends on energy intake).

Biochemical Functions
(a) Cofactor for pyruvate dehydrogenase in the "link reaction" between glycolysis and Krebs Cycle. Involved in energy metabolism from glucose and other carbohydrates.
(b) Cofactor for α-ketoglutarate dehydrogenase
(c) Cofactor for several α-ketoacid dehydrogenases, eg the branched-chain α-ketoacid dehydrogenases involved in amino acid oxidation
(d) Cofactor for transketolase in the Pentose Phosphate Pathway

Diagnostic Tests
(a) Hyperlactataemia especially after a glucose load when pyruvate and lactate (which are immediately upstream of pyruvate dehydrogenase) accumulate.
(b) Measurement of red blood cell transketolase activity in the absence and presence of additional thiamin
Dietary sources: Cereals, pulses, yeast, liver

Deficiency diseases
(a) Associated with alcohol abuse causing Wernicke's encephalopathy and Korsakoff's dementia
(b) Wet beriberi: oedema, cardiovascular disease; and Dry beriberi: neuropathy and muscle wasting

Toxicity   3g/day (variety of clinical signs)

Niacin (Vitamin B₃)

Niacin is a component of the hydrogen carriers, NAD⁺ and NADP⁺. Both have numerous roles in metabolism but NAD⁺ is especially important as a "hydrogen carrier" for ATP production by the respiratory chain, whereas NADPH is very important for biosynthetic reactions. Daily requirement: 6.6 niacin equivalents/1000 kcal

Biochemical function: niacin is a term for nicotinic acid & nicotinamide. A component of NAD⁺ and NADP⁺; and their reduced forms, NADH and NADPH which are involved in numerous metabolic reactions.
NAD⁺ is involved in glycolysis, the oxidation of fatty acids, amino acid oxidation and Krebs Cycle. It is particularly important as a "hydrogen carrier" since oxidation of NADH by the respiratory chain generates ATP. NADP⁺ and its reduced form NADPH⁺ are particularly important in biosynthetic reactions eg lipid synthesis.

Diagnostic test for deficiency: measure the ratio in urine of NMN/pyridone (N'-methylnicotinamide / N'-methyl-2-pyridone-5-carboximide)

Dietary sources: vitamin enriched breakfast cereals, liver, yeast, meat, pulses.
Approximately half daily requirement can be biosynthesised from tryptophan (60 mg of tryptophan ≡ 1 mg niacin).

Deficiency diseases: Pellagra (from the Italian "rough skin") occurs if diet is deficient in BOTH niacin and tryptophan such as maize-based diets (dermatitis, diarrhoea, dementia).

Pharmacology/toxicity: Pharmacological doses (of 2 – 4 g daily) have been used in trials as a hypolipidaemic agent.
Excessive nicotinic acid can cause transient vasodilation with hypotension.

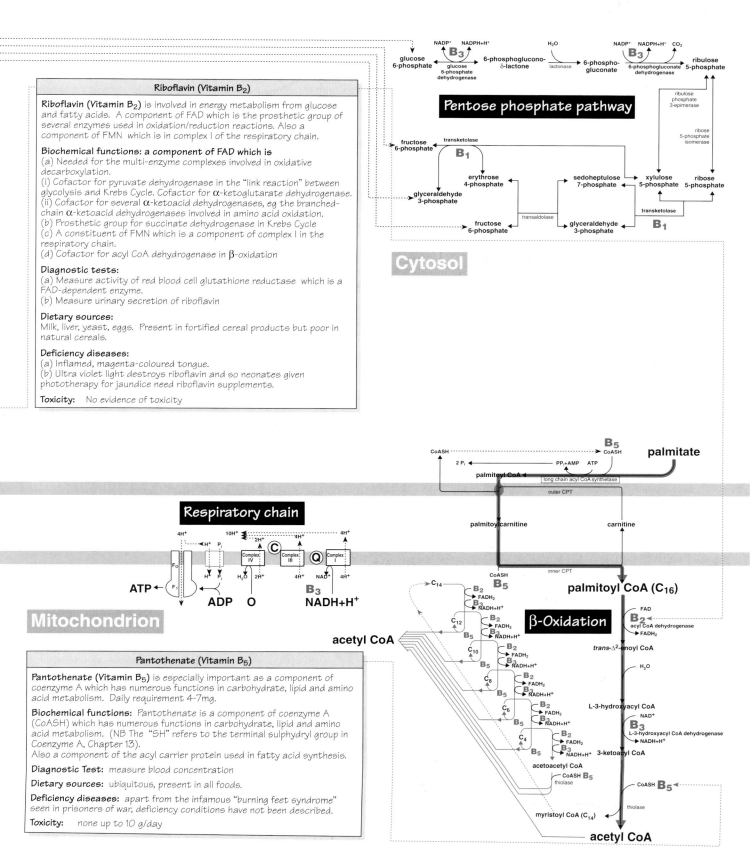

Riboflavin (Vitamin B₂)

Riboflavin (Vitamin B₂) is involved in energy metabolism from glucose and fatty acids. A component of FAD which is the prosthetic group of several enzymes used in oxidation/reduction reactions. Also a component of FMN which is in complex I of the respiratory chain.

Biochemical functions: a component of FAD which is
(a) Needed for the multi-enzyme complexes involved in oxidative decarboxylation.
(i) Cofactor for pyruvate dehydrogenase in the "link reaction" between glycolysis and Krebs Cycle. Cofactor for α-ketoglutarate dehydrogenase.
(ii) Cofactor for several α-ketoacid dehydrogenases, eg the branched-chain α-ketoacid dehydrogenases involved in amino acid oxidation.
(b) Prosthetic group for succinate dehydrogenase in Krebs Cycle
(c) A constituent of FMN which is a component of complex I in the respiratory chain.
(d) Cofactor for acyl CoA dehydrogenase in β-oxidation

Diagnostic tests:
(a) Measure activity of red blood cell glutathione reductase which is a FAD-dependent enzyme.
(b) Measure urinary secretion of riboflavin

Dietary sources:
Milk, liver, yeast, eggs. Present in fortified cereal products but poor in natural cereals.

Deficiency diseases:
(a) Inflamed, magenta-coloured tongue.
(b) Ultra violet light destroys riboflavin and so neonates given phototherapy for jaundice need riboflavin supplements.

Toxicity: No evidence of toxicity

Pantothenate (Vitamin B₅)

Pantothenate (Vitamin B₅) is especially important as a component of coenzyme A which has numerous functions in carbohydrate, lipid and amino acid metabolism. Daily requirement 4-7mg.

Biochemical functions: Pantothenate is a component of coenzyme A (CoASH) which has numerous functions in carbohydrate, lipid and amino acid metabolism. (NB The "SH" refers to the terminal sulphydryl group in Coenzyme A, Chapter 13).
Also a component of the acyl carrier protein used in fatty acid synthesis.

Diagnostic Test: measure blood concentration

Dietary sources: ubiquitous, present in all foods.

Deficiency diseases: apart from the infamous "burning feet syndrome" seen in prisoners of war, deficiency conditions have not been described.

Toxicity: none up to 10 g/day

Figure 55.1 The role of water-soluble vitamins in metabolism.

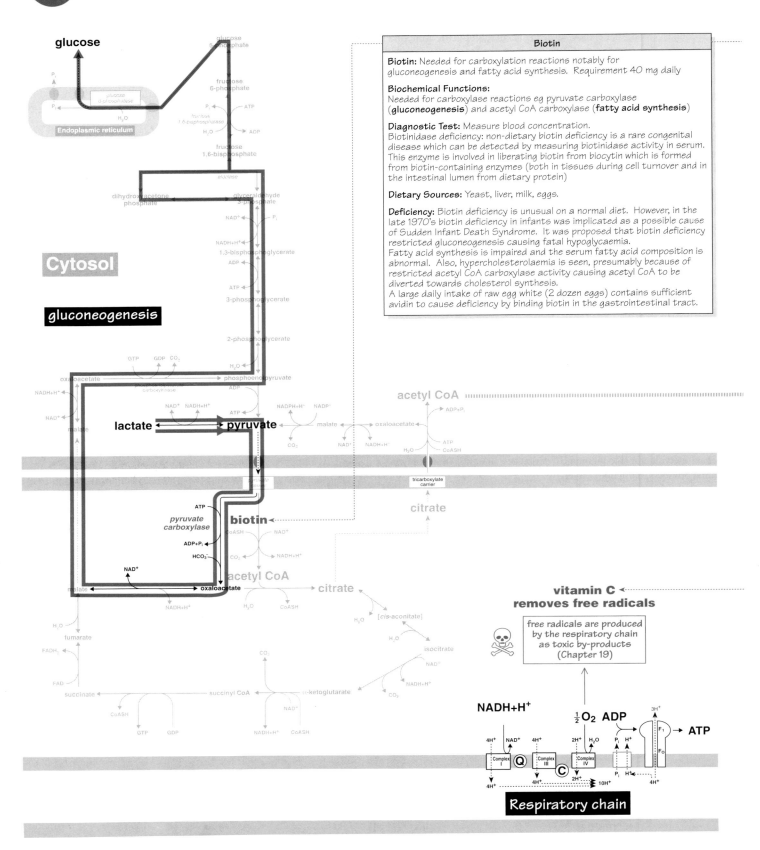

Biotin

Biotin: Needed for carboxylation reactions notably for gluconeogenesis and fatty acid synthesis. Requirement 40 mg daily

Biochemical Functions:
Needed for carboxylase reactions eg pyruvate carboxylase (**gluconeogenesis**) and acetyl CoA carboxylase (**fatty acid synthesis**)

Diagnostic Test: Measure blood concentration.
Biotinidase deficiency: non-dietary biotin deficiency is a rare congenital disease which can be detected by measuring biotinidase activity in serum. This enzyme is involved in liberating biotin from biocytin which is formed from biotin-containing enzymes (both in tissues during cell turnover and in the intestinal lumen from dietary protein)

Dietary Sources: Yeast, liver, milk, eggs.

Deficiency: Biotin deficiency is unusual on a normal diet. However, in the late 1970's biotin deficiency in infants was implicated as a possible cause of Sudden Infant Death Syndrome. It was proposed that biotin deficiency restricted gluconeogenesis causing fatal hypoglycaemia.
Fatty acid synthesis is impaired and the serum fatty acid composition is abnormal. Also, hypercholesterolaemia is seen, presumably because of restricted acetyl CoA carboxylase activity causing acetyl CoA to be diverted towards cholesterol synthesis.
A large daily intake of raw egg white (2 dozen eggs) contains sufficient avidin to cause deficiency by binding biotin in the gastrointestinal tract.

vitamin C ◄
removes free radicals

free radicals are produced by the respiratory chain as toxic by-products (Chapter 19)

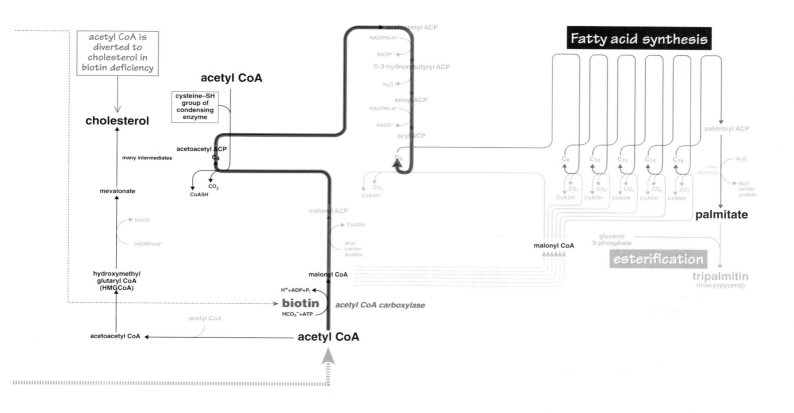

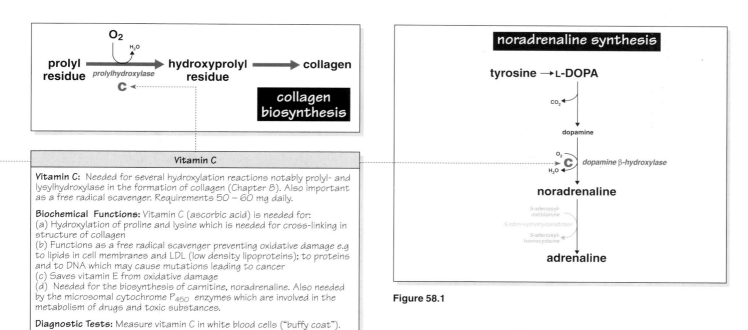

Figure 58.1

Vitamin C

Vitamin C: Needed for several hydroxylation reactions notably prolyl- and lysylhydroxylase in the formation of collagen (Chapter 8). Also important as a free radical scavenger. Requirements 50 – 60 mg daily.

Biochemical Functions: Vitamin C (ascorbic acid) is needed for:
(a) Hydroxylation of proline and lysine which is needed for cross-linking in structure of collagen
(b) Functions as a free radical scavenger preventing oxidative damage e.g to lipids in cell membranes and LDL (low density lipoproteins); to proteins and to DNA which may cause mutations leading to cancer
(c) Saves vitamin E from oxidative damage
(d) Needed for the biosynthesis of carnitine, noradrenaline. Also needed by the microsomal cytochrome P_{450} enzymes which are involved in the metabolism of drugs and toxic substances.

Diagnostic Tests: Measure vitamin C in white blood cells ("buffy coat").

Dietary Sources: Fresh fruit particularly citrus fruits, and vegetables.

Deficiency: Impaired synthesis of collagen leads to scurvy characterised by bleeding gums, bruising and poor wound healing.
Vitamin C supplements improve wound-healing and decrease skin-bruising in some types of Ehlers-Danlos syndrome.

59 Diagnostic clinical chemistry (with Dr JW Wright FRCP, MRCPath)

NB [H^+] indicates proton concentration which is inversely related to pH, (Chapter 1 & 2)

Column headings and reference ranges:

- **Sodium** (135–145 mMol/L)
- **Potassium** (3.5–5.0 mMol/L)
- **Bicarbonate** (23–33 mMol/L)
- **Urea** (3–7 mMol/L or BUN 8–20 mg/dL)
- **Uric acid** reference range – see below
- **Creatinine** (60–120 μMol/L or 0.6-1.3 mg/dL)
- **Glucose** Fasting < 6.0 mMol/L or < 108 mg/dL
- **Phosphate** (0.8–1.4 mMol/L or 2.5–4.3 mg/dL)
- **Calcium** (2.0–2.5 mMol/L or 8-10 mg/dL)
- **Albumin** (30–50 g/L or 3-5 g/dL)
- **Total cholesterol** (target <4.0 mMol/L or < 155mg/dL [for patients on treatment])
- **Triglycerides (triacylglycerols)** (< 1.5 mMol/L or < 133 mg/dL)
- **Alkaline phosphatase** Check local reference range
- **Bilirubin** (< 20 μMol/L or < 1.2 mg/dL)
- **γ-Glutamyltransferase** (γ-GT) Check local reference range
- **ALT** (Alanine aminotransferase) Check local reference range
- **LDH** (Lactate dehydrogenase) Check local reference range
- **CK** (Creatine kinase) Check local reference range
- **Free thyroxine** (7–25 pMol/L or 0.5–2 ng/dL)
- **TSH** (Thyroid stimulating hormone) 0.3–5.0 mU/L

	Sodium	Potassium	Bicarbonate	Urea	Uric acid	Creatinine	Glucose	Phosphate	Calcium	Albumin	Total cholesterol	Triglycerides	Alkaline phosphatase	Bilirubin	γ-GT	ALT	LDH	CK	Free thyroxine	TSH	Other tests and comments
Kidney disease																					
Acute nephritis	N↓	↑	N↓	↑	E↑	↑		N↑													Proteinuria, haematuria, casts, ASO titre ↑, complement ↓.
Acute renal failure	N↓	⇑	↓	⇑	E↑	⇑		↑	N↓	N↓											Urinary Na ↓ in pre-renal failure.
Chronic renal failure	N	⇑	↓	⇑	E↑	⇑		⬆	↓↑	N↓	↑	↑	N↑								If calcium is raised, possibility of primary tertiary hyperparathyroidism.
Nephrotic syndrome	N↓	N↑	N↓	↗		↗			↓	⬇	↑								E↓	N	Heavy proteinuria. Differential protein clearance useful in assessing prognosis.
Renal calculi					N↑				N↑												Check urine calcium, urate, oxalate. Rare possibility of cystinuria.
Liver disease																					
Acute hepatitis				N↓						N			↑	⇑	↑	⬆	↑				Check viral status (A, B and C). Urine bilirubin ↑ especially during recovery phase, occasionally anicteric. Check toxins.
Acute hepatic necrosis				↓			↓			N			↑	↑	↑	⬆	↑				Prothrombin time prolonged. Bilirubin rises and enzymes fall as disease progresses.
Chronic hepatitis: persistent				N			N			N			N↑	N↑	N↑	↑	N↑				Check hep B antigen.
Chronic hepatitis: active				N↓			N			N↓			↑	↑	↑	⇑	↑				IgG ↑, ANF and smooth muscle antibodies may be +ve.
Primary biliary cirrhosis										N↓	↑		⬆	↗	⬆	N↑	↑				Mitochondrial antibodies +ve, IgM↑, caeruloplasmin ↑.
Portal cirrhosis	↓	N↓		↓			N		E↓	⬇			N↑	N↑	↑	↑	N↑				Prothrombin time prolonged, diffuse ↑ γ globulins, urinary urobilinogen ↑. Check for Wilson's disease (serum copper), haemochromatosis (serum iron), α-1-antitrypsin deficiency.
Extrahepatic obstruction										N	↑		⇑	⇑	↑	N↑					Urinary bilirubin ↑.
Infiltration/invasion										N			↑	N↑	↑	N↑					In localised liver disease, γ-GT and Alk Phos may be ↑ without jaundice.
Haemolytic jaundice								N↑		N			N	↑	N	N	↑				Unconjugated bilirubin ↑, reticulocytes ↑, urinary bilirubin –ve, urinary urobilinogen ↑.
Alcohol abuse					↑		↓↑			N↓		↑	N↑	N↑	↑	N↑		R↑			Consider measuring blood alcohol. MCV ↑. NB Check for hypoglycaemia in alcohol coma especially in children.
Cardiovascular disease																					
Myocardial infarction																↑	⇑	⇑			Measure troponin I (or CK–MB) in acute situation. Sequence of enzyme elevation is: CK, AST, LDH
Cardiac failure	N↓		N↑	N↑		N↑									N↑	N↑	N↑	N			Raised enzymes may indicate ischaemic hepatitis.
Gastro-intestinal disease																					
Vomiting (with water replacement)	↓	↓	↑	N					N	N											Dilutional hyponatraemia.
Vomiting (without water replacement)	↑	N↓	↑	↑					↑	↑											Changes are due to dehydration and chloride depletion.
Bleeding	N	N		↑		N															Urea is elevated especially in upper GI tract bleeding.
Malabsorption									↓	↓			N↑								Faecal fat ↑, faecal elastase ↓. Folate, B_{12}, and Ca may be ↓. Prothrombin time may be prolonged. Measure endomysial antibodies for celiac disease.
Inflammatory bowel disease	N↓	N↓		N↓		N			↓	↓			N↑			N↑					May show some features of malabsorption.
Diarrhoea		↓	↓	N↑		N				N↑											Changes are seen in prolonged diarrhoea.
Acute pancreatitis	N↓	N					↑		↓	↓		↑		N↑	N↑						Serum amylase ↑ for 2–3 days. Serum methaemalbumin ↑ in severe cases.

Respiratory disease

Condition	Findings
Acute respiratory failure	$pO_2 \downarrow$, $pCO_2 \uparrow$, $[H^+]\uparrow$, $pH \downarrow$ Uncompensated respiratory acidosis
Chronic respiratory failure	$pO_2 \downarrow$, $pCO_2 \uparrow$, $[H^+]$ N/$\uparrow$, pH N/$\downarrow$ Compensated respiratory acidosis

Bone and joint disease

Osteoporosis	Diagnosis depends on bone mineral density scan rather than biochemistry
Rickets & osteomalacia	Vitamin D $\downarrow$
Paget's disease	Calcium may increase with immobilisation.
Primary hyperparathyroidism	PTH inappropriately high. Steroid suppression test: calcium remains high.
Hypercalcaemia of malignancy	Steroid suppression test: calcium usually falls. PTH is not raised.
Gout	Exclude renal dysfunction and diuretic treatment as cause of hyperuricaemia.
Myeloma	Paraprotein band on electrophoresis. Confirm and characterise with immune electrophoresis; plasma cells $\uparrow$ in bone marrow, Bence-Jones proteinuria

Endocrine diseases

Condition	Findings
Diabetes mellitus	Diagnostic criteria: fasting blood glucose > 7 mMol/L and/or 2 hours post 75g glucose load > 11.1 mMol/L
Diabetic ketoacidosis	Glucosuria and ketonuria. Blood $[H^+]\uparrow$, $pH \downarrow$. Creatinine may be spuriously $\uparrow$ if measured by Jaffe method. NB Total body potassium and sodium are low
Hypothyroidism	TSH is used as first-line test for thyroid disorders
Hyperthyroidism	TSH unresponsive to TRH.
Addison's disease (adrenal insufficiency)	Do synacthen test (if possible) before treating with steroids. Plasma cortisol $\downarrow$ and unresponsive to synacthen. Plasma ACTH $\uparrow$
Cushing's syndrome	Plasma and 24h urine cortisol $\uparrow$. Cortisol not suppressed by dexamethasone. Loss of diurnal variation of cortisol. Plasma ACTH inappropriately $\uparrow$ in pituitary Cushing's, very $\uparrow$ in ectopic ACTH, suppressed in adrenal Cushing's
Conn's syndrome	Plasma renin $\downarrow$, aldosterone $\uparrow$.
Diabetes insipidus	Water deprivation test: polyuria persists; urine does not concentrate
Inappropriate ADH (SIADH)	Urine osmolality less than maximally dilute; urine sodium inappropriately $\uparrow$. Exclude adrenal insufficiency, renal failure and diuretic therapy.

TSH Elevated in neonates (up to 40 mU/L)

Free thyroxine Non-specific decrease seen in many ill patients. Free T_3 also available.

CK Originates from cardiac muscle, skeletal & smooth muscle and brain. Isoenzyme measurements used, particularly CK-MB in myocardial infarction

LDH Originates from liver, heart, skeletal muscle, red cells and kidney

ALT Moderately raised in obesity and metabolic syndrome. Marker for non-alcoholic fatty liver

γ-Glutamyltransferase (γGT) Increased with alcohol abuse and by other enzyme inducers e.g. phenytoin, barbiturates and abdominal obesity.

Bilirubin Gilbert's disease is a common cause of benign unconjugated hyperbilirubinaemia

Alkaline phosphatase Isoenzyme measurements may help to distinguish between bone, liver, intestinal and placental fractions. Raised during fracture healing, late pregnancy and in children during rapid growth.

Triglycerides (triacylglycerols) Fasting specimen recommended.

Cholesterol See British Joint Societies Lipid Guidelines (2004)

Sodium Large alterations are usually due to changed water balance. Often non-specifically $\downarrow$ in ill patients.

Potassium Spuriously elevated in unseparated or haemolysed specimens

Bicarbonate If the results are grossly abnormal check blood gases and $[H^+]$ (or pH)

Urea Increased in dehydration, but clinical signs are of more value. Varies with dietary protein.

Uric acid Varies with dietary protein. Normal range: 0.12–0.42 mMol/l (male & post-menopausal female), 0.12–0.36 mMol/l (pre-menopausal female).

Creatinine Creatinine clearance usually gives no additional information

Glucose Timing with respect to meals is critical.

Phosphate Falls after carbohydrate meals. Elevated in haemolysed/unseparated specimens

Calcium Total serum calcium related to albumin levels; adjusted by calculating "corrected calcium". Avoid venous stasis (falsely high values)

Albumin Many laboratory methods tend to overestimate low values

---

Key

N	Normal
N (arrow down)	Normal or low
N (arrow up)	Normal or high
(up arrow)	High to very high
(down arrow)	Low to very low
(double arrow)	Low or high
(down arrow)	Very low
(up arrow)	Very high
E	Epiphenomenon, low. Not of diagnostic value.
E	Epiphenomenon, high. Not of diagnostic value.
R	Rare, high. An uncommon association.
R	Rare, low. Not of diagnostic value.
(arrow)	Tends to rise with progression of disease.

This simple guide cannot include the innumerable variables which influence biochemical tests and their interpretation. It should be used with caution, discretion and in conjunction with the clinical features and other tests which contribute to the final diagnosis.

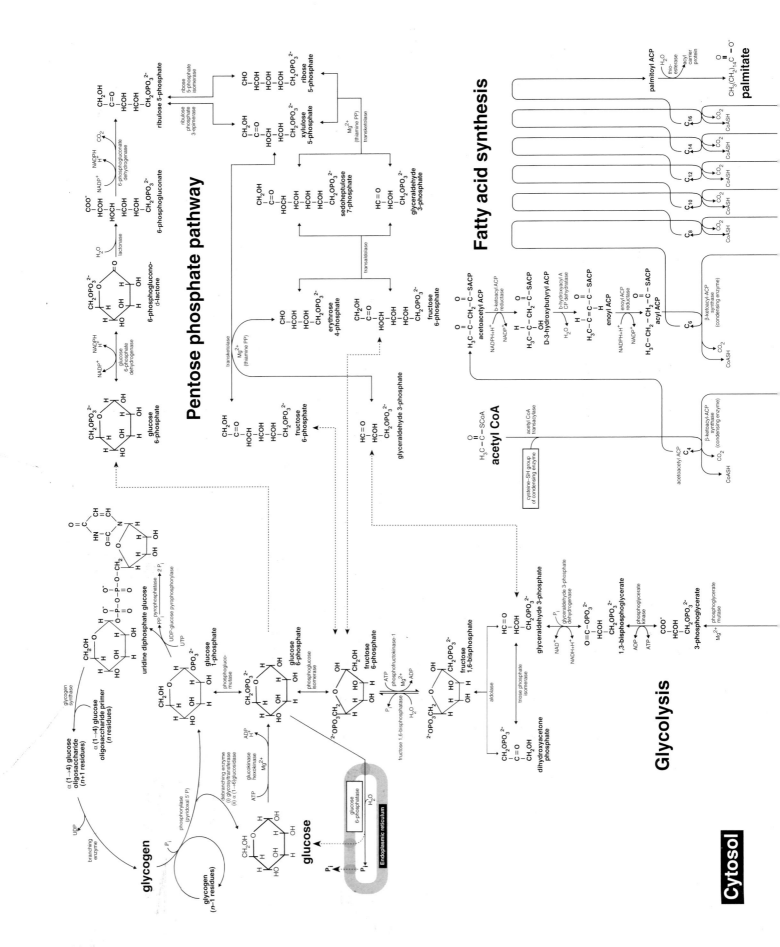